CASE STUDIES IN

Population and Community Health Management

CASE STUDIES IN

Population and Community Health Management

Connie J. Evashwick ▪ Jason S. Turner ▪ Editors

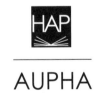

AUPHA

Health Administration Press, Chicago, Illinois

Association of University Programs in Health Administration, Washington, DC

24   23   22   21   20   5   4   3   2   1

Library of Congress Cataloging-in-Publication Data

Names: Evashwick, Connie, editor. | Turner, Jason S., editor. | Health Administration Press, publisher. | Association of University Programs in Health Administration, issuing body.
Title: Case studies in population and community health management / [edited by] Connie J. Evashwick, Jason S. Turner.
Description: Chicago, Illinois ; Washington, DC : HAP/AUPHA, [2020] | Includes bibliographical references. | Summary: "The cases in this book emphasize the application of healthcare management principles and skills across institutional boundaries to effectively manage the health status of a population or community"— Provided by publisher.
Identifiers: LCCN 2019033887 (print) | LCCN 2019033888 (ebook) | ISBN 9781640551251 (hardcover ; alk. paper) | ISBN 9781640551268 (ebook) | ISBN 9781640551275 (ebook) | ISBN 9781640551282 (epub) | ISBN 9781640551299 (mobi)
Subjects: MESH: Community Health Planning | Population Health Management | Community Health Services—organization & administration | Needs Assessment | Organizational Case Studies | United States
Classification: LCC RA418.3.U6 (print) | LCC RA418.3.U6 (ebook) | NLM WA 546 AA1 | DDC 362.10973—dc23
LC record available at https://lccn.loc.gov/2019033887
LC ebook record available at https://lccn.loc.gov/2019033888
The paper used in this publication meets the minimum requirements of American National Standard for Information Sciences—Permanence of Paper for Printed Library Materials, ANSI Z39.48-1984. ∞™

Acquisitions editor: Janet Davis; Project manager: Michael Noren; Cover designer: James Slate; Layout: Integra

Found an error or a typo? We want to know! Please email it to hapbooks@ache.org, mentioning the book's title and putting "Book Error" in the subject line.

For photocopying and copyright information, please contact Copyright Clearance Center at www.copyright.com or at (978) 750-8400.

Health Administration Press   Association of University Programs
A division of the Foundation of the American   in Health Administration
   College of Healthcare Executives   1730 M Street, NW
300 S. Riverside Plaza, Suite 1900   Suite 407
Chicago, IL 60606-6698   Washington, DC 20036
(312) 424-2800   (202) 763-7283

To my family, friends, and colleagues who have taught me over the years about community of residence and community of spirit.
CE

To my wife and children, who show me abundant patience and love.
JT

BRIEF CONTENTS

DETAILED CONTENTS

ACKNOWLEDGMENTS

We would like to thank all of the authors who were willing to trail-blaze in writing cases for a new book. We'd also like to thank the colleagues who reviewed various sections, specifically Ms. Sandra Duncan, Mr. Daniel Fahey, Dr. Todd Grant, Mr. Keith Jennings, Dr. Michael Peddecord, Mr. Ryan Schiel, and Ms. Jillian Warriner, as well as Dr. Judith Connell, who reviewed the entire book.

The need for a book of case studies on community and population health arose because of the vision of Dr. Robert E. Burke and the support of the leadership, faculty, and students of the Executive MHA Program of George Washington University. Our colleagues at Health Administration Press have been terrific, especially Ms. Janet Davis, in encouraging us to persevere with this work, and Mr. Michael Noren, who did a superb job of editing. Our deepest thanks to Ms. Elizabeth Evashwick, JD, and Mr. Alex Henderson, who assisted with compiling the many pieces of the manuscript.

Most of all, we would like to thank all of the healthcare administrators, clinicians, academicians, individuals, and families who are advancing the concepts of community health and population health. To paraphrase esteemed educator Dr. John Gardiner, "Change always looks chaotic when you are in the middle of it; clarity only appears once you've come out the other side." Eventually, we will improve the health status of the population and create a health system that promotes the health of communities and all who are part of them. Thank you for joining us on the journey.

Connie and Jason

INTRODUCTION: MANAGING "BEYOND THE WALLS"

The purpose of this book is to use the analysis of practical cases to educate health-care leaders about managing the health of populations and communities. Historically, healthcare executives have been taught how to lead and manage *within* their organizations, with minimal attention to external relationships. However, in today's health landscape—with evolving payment models and growing recognition of the importance of social determinants—this kind of internal orientation is no longer sufficient. The ability to manage "beyond the walls" of the institution has become essential to the success of any healthcare leader.

Today's healthcare leaders must understand the communities they serve, the special populations for which they assume risk, and the other organizations along the continuum of care that provide or pay for services. The cases in this book emphasize the application of healthcare management principles and skills across institutional boundaries to effectively manage the health status of a population or community.

Defining *Population Health*, *Community Health*, and *Public Health*

The concepts of population health, community health, and public health are closely intertwined, but the terms are not synonymous. An important task for a healthcare executive is to understand the distinctions between the terms and the implications for effective management.

Although consensus on these terms' precise meanings is lacking, this section will propose definitions to be used in analyzing the book's cases. We offer these definitions with the understanding that good managers will see beyond the verbiage to analyze situations and propose realistic and measurable approaches based on the desired goals and objectives. Regardless of the phrasing, common management principles apply.

Population Health
Kindig and Stoddart (2003, 381) defined *population health* as "the health outcomes of a group of individuals, including the distribution of such outcomes within the group, and the factors affecting those outcomes." This definition has been adopted by the National Academy of Sciences Roundtable on Population Health Improvement (2019).

The concept of population health implies both a measurable numerator and a measurable denominator, and it incorporates the ability to measure changes over time. Populations can be subgroups within communities, can encompass multiple communities, or can cut across community lines.

Population health management is a more explicit term that describes active interventions to control the health status or healthcare utilization of a defined and identifiable group of individuals. For example, a managed care company might have a population health management program in which it provides all of its members who have a diagnosis of diabetes with a cellular phone loaded with an app that sends daily reminders about monitoring their hemoglobin A1c level (and perhaps even reports the results to the doctor's office automatically). The company would have the denominator of all enrollees, the numerator of all enrollees with a diagnosis of diabetes, and a way of monitoring the health status of the individuals with the app. It would therefore be able to determine whether the app made a difference in utilization of healthcare services or in the long-term health status of individuals or the aggregate population.

Community Health

Community health is a much broader term than *population health*, and it can be ambiguous. For the purpose of these cases, *community health* can be defined as the health of a group of individuals who share a bond of geography, culture, race, ethnicity, language, sexual orientation, pastime passion, or another common characteristic (Merriam-Webster 2019).

In many instances, community health offers no ability to measure either the denominator or the numerator. As a result, the success of a community health initiative in attaining its goals and objectives can be hard to demonstrate—which can be a challenge when trying to secure institutional commitment or resources for an intervention. Regardless, improving the health of populations and individuals requires improving the health of the communities in which they reside.

An example of a community health program might be a booth at a health fair at a local Catholic church at which a home care agency provides free screening for diabetes. The agency might have selected this approach because it knows that many members of the parish are Hispanic and that Hispanics have demonstrated high rates of diabetes and undiagnosed diabetes. The agency would have no idea how many people saw notices about the health fair (other than estimating based on the parish's total membership or the fair's total attendance), but it would have a record of how many people it screened and how many tested positive. Hopefully, the agency would also know how to contact those individuals whose test results called for active follow-up.

Public Health

Charles Winslow (1920, 30) defined *public health* broadly as "the science and art of preventing disease, prolonging life, and promoting physical health and efficiency" through organized community efforts and informed choices of society, organizations, communities, and individuals. In this book, we will use the phrase *public health* in the specific context of the public health structure of the United States.

The US public health system includes a number of government agencies that have been created to fulfill the provisions of public health legislation and to carry out the government's role in safeguarding the public. This bureaucracy includes the Centers for Disease Control and Prevention, a federal agency; departments of health for every state and territory; and local health departments (LHDs). Funds for essential public health functions flow from the federal government to states and from states to local agencies.

Most health departments serve a designated geographic area, with all residents of that area considered to be the department's responsibility. For program purposes, the denominator can usually be regarded as the number of residents of a department's geography, based on the most recent census count. However, complications arise when public health programs affect residents in adjacent areas or do not reach all residents within the designated area.

An example of a public health approach to diabetes control might involve a local radio broadcast of a series of public service announcements (PSAs) that encourage women who are pregnant and have certain symptoms to be screened for gestational diabetes at their LHD or by their own physician. The LHD would know the total number of people in its catchment area, and it might also keep count of the number of new pregnant patients who come to the department's clinics for screening within a given period after the PSA broadcast. However, the LHD would not know the total number of pregnant women in its catchment area, the number of people who heard and remembered the announcement, or the number of women who were screened—unless it made a special effort to gather such information.

Overlapping Functions

As is evident from these examples, public health, community health, and population health programs often overlap, with multiple interventions reaching the same individuals. Conversely, public health, community health, and population health programs may occur simultaneously, with similar long-term purposes, yet remain distinct—for instance, by sending out different messages about the same condition or having different interventions aimed at the same long-term outcome.

The federal government and various private organizations have made great strides in setting up databases that collect evidence about the impact of certain interventions for specific populations (see, for example, the Community Guide, at www.thecommunityguide.org). The task of the healthcare executive is to sort out which programs apply to which target audiences and for what short-term and long-term outcomes. Ideally, health promotion programs and population health management interventions can then be organized to complement rather than compete with one another. Desired improvements in the health status of the community can be better achieved and sustained by collaborative efforts than by individual programs, and use of resources can be maximized.

Whether a program is considered "population," "community," or "public" health, common managerial principles apply. This book aims to provide a foundation for understanding why and how to apply these principles "beyond the walls" of a single organization.

Trends

Several disparate trends are converging to amplify the importance of community and population health to the field of healthcare management. A critical underlying premise: Each of these factors plays out differently from one community to another, and thus no single way of managing will be universally appropriate. Understanding the key overarching concepts and developing the ability to apply them locally are essential for a healthcare executive's success.

The concept of the Triple Aim—first introduced by the Institute for Healthcare Improvement (IHI) in 2007 (Berwick, Nolan, and Whittington 2008)—has brought increasing attention to the health status of populations. The three components of the Triple Aim are cost, the patient experience of care, and population health (IHI 2019). The purpose of the Triple Aim is to convey, in easily repeatable terms, the three different spheres that need to be addressed to make the nation's healthcare system effective and sustainable. Whereas experts in healthcare management and policy (HMP) have long been familiar with the challenges associated with cost and quality, the inclusion of population health as part of the troika was a new development that helped bridge HMP with knowledge that had been generated in the field of public health. Healthcare executives gained a better understanding of the impact of the community on individuals' health.

A related trend involves the growing recognition of the degree to which social determinants of health (SDoH) shape an individual's health status. The field of public health has spent decades compiling concrete evidence about the health effects of factors external to the individual. Today, it is often said that people's zip codes are as important to their health as their genetic codes, reflecting the growing acknowledgment of the health impact of "where one lives, learns, works, plays, and prays." As these factors are increasingly taken into account, interventions to improve health status have expanded beyond the one-on-one patient–provider relationship to target broad communities and specific population groups. A definitive statement on the SDoH has been provided by the World Health Organization (WHO 2019).

In addition, ongoing efforts to control healthcare costs at the national level have led to new and revised payment models. The use of bundled and capitated payment models, as well as links of payment to performance, have further brought the healthcare status of populations to the forefront. Many of these models incorporate funding based on populations rather than on care for individuals, as well as payment for a set of services rather than distinct fees for itemized procedures (Centers for Medicare & Medicaid Services 2019). The capitated systems of the health maintenance organizations (HMOs) of the 1970s and 1980s, which gave hope for more efficient use of resources, are being revisited, with a focus on revising rules to ameliorate the flaws that haunted the earlier HMO models. Some risk-adjusted payment models require that providers and payers consider a target audience of communities or populations rather than individuals. The movement toward population-based health is not limited to the United States; it is also global (Aaronson et al. 2019).

The concept of *quality* continues to evolve as an essential, distinct, measurable component of healthcare, with population health now recognized as a key aspect. The National Committee for Quality Assurance (NCQA 2018) has launched a new certification on population health management.

Finally, information systems have expanded, big data have become more readily available, and the science of informatics in healthcare has grown into its own specialty. Information systems and the accompanying technologies enable individuals to track their own data and institutions to compile these data. Hospitals and physicians have implemented electronic health records that record detailed patient information over time, and health and health-related agencies throughout a community have agreed to share data that enhance the quality of patient care. Data are now available, as never before, to understand the health of communities and to manage the health of population subgroups.

Using This Book

The case study approach in this book is based on pedagogical principles applicable to adult learners. The guiding theory is that adults learn more by analyzing problems, finding data, applying management theories, and proposing solutions than by having information dictated to them. The cases in this book present opportunities for students of all healthcare disciplines who take management courses, or for healthcare executives, to analyze real-world situations, find and apply data, and pose practical approaches to address the issues presented. Challenges and solutions should be supported with data. No single answer is expected. Critical thinking and robust discussion are desired.

Competencies and Learning Objectives
The overarching theme of the cases is the application of generic management skills to the healthcare system in the United States. Cases are intended to arm students with practical skills—identified here as *competencies*—as well as didactic knowledge, or *learning objectives.*

The learning objectives are broad in scope and might emphasize acquisition of didactic knowledge as a prerequisite or foundation for application. The competencies are drawn from those prioritized by health professions accrediting agencies, including the Council on Education for Public Health (CEPH), the Commission on Accreditation of Healthcare Management Education (CAHME), and the Certified Health Education Specialist (CHES) credentialing body.

The cases can be distinguished from other forms of healthcare management literature in that they present a healthcare system that extends beyond the walls of a given organization, encompassing all of the service providers, payers, and coordinating health and social service agencies in a community and extending to the social determinants of health.

Instructors teaching these cases can adapt them to meet the accreditation requirements, pedagogical frameworks, or syllabus templates applicable to their individual program or institution. The learning objectives identified for each case should be useful regardless of which framework or accreditation body governs a given program. From an applied perspective, good management skills are equally relevant to all disciplines.

Overall, the cases in this book are intended to help students master the knowledge and skills needed to do the following:

- Characterize the residents of a community.
- Analyze the components of the healthcare system of a community, which includes identifying stakeholders.
- Apply fundamental management skills to community and population health; such skills span the areas of strategic planning, human resources, information systems, finance, marketing, communications, and project management, among others.
- Define and differentiate *community health*, *population health*, and *public health*.
- Apply the social determinants of health and Ecological Model of Health concepts.
- Analyze the health status of a defined population.
- Guide the conduct of a community health needs assessment.
- Develop a community health improvement plan.
- Assess the power structure of a community.
- Contrast collective impact with collaborative and individual initiatives.
- Evaluate the roles of state and local public health departments in influencing the health status of a community.
- Measure change in the health status of a community or population over time.
- Evaluate the impact of specific interventions on the health status of a population over time.
- Analyze the financial implications for healthcare institutions of managing the health of a defined population.
- Explain the information systems necessary to monitor and manage the health and service utilization of a population across settings and over time.
- Differentiate the methods to influence the health of a defined population from the methods to influence the health of a community.

- Contrast care of an individual patient by a single provider with care provided by a comprehensive continuum of care.
- Analyze a communications strategy designed for a specific target audience.
- Evaluate the effectiveness of communications techniques designed for population health management.
- Specify the elements essential to sustaining a community or population health program over time.
- Analyze the business case for a health organization to be involved with its community.
- Analyze the business case for a health organization to be involved with managing the health of a defined population.

Each of the book's cases presents an *overarching theme*—however, this theme should not preclude students from exploring other related topics.

The Cases

Each case is a stand-alone example of a real-world situation, and each requires understanding of a target audience and stakeholders, analysis of the problem(s), a search for relevant data to inform the issue, critical thinking to identify action options, and criteria with which to make decisions. An evidence-based approach includes projecting SMART objectives—that is, objectives that are specific, measurable, attainable, relevant, and time bound—and evaluation with measurable targets of success.

Each case is framed with a *management challenge*. Students are asked to respond to a specific task, drawing from the background information presented. However, many secondary topics are woven into the cases, proffering opportunities for students to pursue additional information about health conditions, target audiences, or management applications. Lists of questions—consisting of fact and data analysis questions as well as discussion questions—are provided at the end of each case. The questions, which are intended to spark analysis and exploration, can be supplemented based on students' interests and the pedagogical approach of the course or curriculum.

The cases present a three-dimensional matrix of management skills, health topics, and population subgroups. Management skills essential for healthcare are the primary focus of the book. Not all salient health topics or population subgroups are included. Readers are encouraged to be thorough in analyzing the problems important for every community and to be creative in finding ways to solve them.

Timeliness and Ethics

The cases in this book represent both real-world communities and organizations and ones that are fabricated but based on the authors' real experience. All real organizations have given permission to have their information included. We ask for readers' appreciation for the sensitivity of information, both that which is presented here and that which can be found on the internet or via other sources. If information has changed or a community context has evolved, readers can regard such developments as part of real-time management, and they can modify the case accordingly.

Similarly, to emphasize the importance of acting on evidence, we have sought to provide data in both hard and fluid formats. Although we have tried to include information that will remain accessible via the internet, it is possible that, over time, some information might cease to be available. We apologize if this occurs. Our hope is that students and instructors will be able to find new and updated data and real-time cases that present similar histories and provocative futures.

The underlying purpose of this book is to apply management concepts to contemporary healthcare problems, thereby pushing the field to embrace community and population health while maintaining excellence in providing services for individual health. Although this shift in perspective can be challenging, we hope these cases will make the change meaningful and rewarding.

References

Aaronson, W., E. Averett, T. T. H. Wan, B. Jordin, A. M. Malik, and A. Pilyavskyy. 2019. "Managing the Health of Populations." In *The Global Healthcare Manager: Competencies, Concepts, and Skills*, edited by M. Counte, B. Ramirez, D. J. West Jr., and W. Aaronson, 421–42. Chicago: Health Administration Press.

Berwick, D. M., T. W. Nolan, and J. Whittington. 2008. "The Triple Aim: Care, Health, and Cost." *Health Affairs*. Published May/June. www.healthaffairs.org/doi/full/10.1377/hlthaff.27.3.759.

Centers for Medicare & Medicaid Services (CMS). 2019. "About the CMS Innovation Center." Accessed June 28. https://innovation.cms.gov/About/.

Institute for Healthcare Improvement (IHI). 2019. "The IHI Triple Aim." Accessed June 28. www.ihi.org/Engage/Initiatives/TripleAim/Pages/default.aspx.

Kindig, D., and G. Stoddart. 2003. "What Is Population Health?" *American Journal of Public Health* 93 (3): 380–83.

Merriam-Webster. 2019. "Community." Accessed June 28. www.merriam-webster.com/dictionary/community.

National Academy of Sciences Roundtable on Population Health Improvement. 2019. "Roundtable on Population Health Improvement." Accessed June 28. http://nationalacademies.org/HMD/Activities/PublicHealth/PopulationHealthImprovementRT.aspx.

National Committee for Quality Assurance (NCQA). 2018. "NCQA Launches New Population Health Management Programs." Published December 10. www.ncqa.org/news/ncqa-launches-new-population-health-management-programs/.

Winslow, C.-E. A. 1920. "The Untilled Fields of Public Health." *Science* 51 (1306): 23–33.

World Health Organization (WHO). 2019. "The Determinants of Health." Accessed June 28. www.who.int/hia/evidence/doh/en/.

Instructor Resources

This book's Instructor Resources include teaching tips for cases; assignments, both individual and group, for each case; definitions of key terms; and a sample syllabus.

For the most up-to-date information about this book and its Instructor Resources, go to ache.org/HAP and browse for the book's title, author name, or order code (2402I).

This book's Instructor Resources are available to instructors who adopt this book for use in their course. For access information, please email hapbooks@ache.org.

UNDERSTANDING A COMMUNITY

A community consists of individuals, families, groups, social networks, and an array of public and private institutions. For a healthcare executive to manage healthcare in a community, an understanding of the residents, institutions, and stakeholders within that community is essential.

Characterizing a Community

A community can be described in terms of the characteristics of its residents, as well as by an array of factors within the environment, ranging from physical characteristics (e.g., air quality, walkability) to policies and regulations (e.g., nonsmoking ordinances). The Ecological Model of Health suggests several major categories of factors to be considered when describing a community and its health status (McElroy et al. 1988).

The first step is to define "the community." Each community is unique and thus has its own definition. A "community" might be defined by geography (e.g., all residents within a given set of zip codes), by age (e.g., a senior living community), religion (e.g., people attending a particular church), or ethnicity (e.g., people of Hispanic descent).

The residents of a community can be described by a variety of demographic, economic, social, and other inherent or acquired characteristics. Various data sets provide information about communities in the United States, and many offer information about health behaviors and health status in particular. When existing data are not sufficient to address a given issue, organizations can gather additional data themselves. To obtain a comprehensive picture of overall community health, general community demographic and economic data may be combined with patient data from healthcare providers; enrollee data from insurers; data about environmental factors; and primary data collected through surveys, interviews, or focus groups.

Benchmarks and standards are available for many health behaviors and conditions, and they can serve as the basis for community-level goals, as well as goals for individual patients. The US Department of Health and Human Services (2019), for instance, maintains a set of targets for priority health conditions in its Healthy People series (www.healthypeople.gov), which is updated each decade. Similarly, the County Health Rankings & Roadmaps (2019) offers a data bank (www.countyhealthrankings. org) through which a county can compare its standing across a number of measures with other counties in its state, or throughout the nation.

Given the number of data sets available—and their growing sophistication—we have a wealth of evidence with which to evaluate the health status of communities and the interventions that affect them. Case 1 of this book focuses on describing the residents of a community, with a particular emphasis on using data, finding relevant data sets, and identifying benchmarks and standards.

Community Health Systems

Community assets are the organizational, physical, financial, political, and social resources that contribute to the health and well-being of a community. Among the most important of these assets is the community's health system, which consists of health organizations and providers, together with related services and organizations. Many of the cases in this book involve identifying the component entities of a community's health system, analyzing the relationships among them, and evaluating the power structure.

Health organizations include hospitals, community clinics, home care agencies, nursing homes, day care centers, dialysis centers, physical therapy clinics, mobile labs, pharmacies, and hearing aid and optical retailers, among many others. Providers include individual physician practices, medical groups, therapists, dentists, nurses, and practitioners working either independently or for formal organizations. Payers include government systems (e.g., Medicare, Medicaid) and private insurers. Support services range from transportation systems for older people to school clinics to water treatment plants. The ways these myriad elements operate vary from one community to another and for specific subsets of the population.

Relationships among these entities vary as well. Some organizations might work well together and exchange client referrals; others might be totally unaware that a particular service even exists in the community. Direct and indirect services may be integrated into a comprehensive continuum of care, or they may function entirely independently. Community-wide information systems, such as 211, may link information about clients even when the service agency staffs do not know one another.

The power structure may differ from one community to another, even if two communities have the same list of organizations. A number of scholars have sought to examine the nature of power. The bases of power proposed by French and Raven (1959)—reward, coercion, legitimate, expert, and referent—can be useful in analyzing relationships among organizations and understanding the public's perception of the organizations serving the community.

Community Asset Mapping

Community asset mapping (CAM) is the process of identifying and characterizing the assets of a community that serve a particular target audience, are based in a defined geographic area, or relate to specific programs of an organization. The purposes of CAM include the following: to enable organizations to determine which entities offer complementary services to their own clients, to identify organizations that might be potential partners, to find organizations with whom data sharing might enhance the quality or efficiency of client care, to recognize gaps in service, and to be alert for potential competitors.

The steps in CAM as it pertains to a specific subset of the population are as follows:

1. Identify the target population being served.
2. Analyze the health and related needs of the target population.
3. Catalog the local organizations that serve this population.
4. Characterize these organizations according to the following:
   - Geographic location
   - Referral patterns/networks
   - Capacity and staff availability
   - Cost of services and payment sources accepted
   - Quality measures
   - Communication mechanisms
   - Potential for collaboration or competition

Information about community assets can come from all types of stakeholders: patients and their families, healthcare staff, physicians, community foundations, board members, local chamber of commerce members, local healthcare professionals associations, and others. Surveys of representatives from each group, or key informant interviews with a select number of individuals, can provide a wealth of information.

Case 2 includes CAM as an important step in the process of developing a new clinic for seniors. CAM can be similarly useful in other situations where an organization seeks to improve quality of care for its clients, improve efficiency of its business operations, or develop a strategic plan for the future.

Community Benefit

The term *community benefit* refers to the idea that a nonprofit hospital must contribute to its community, presumably in an amount equivalent to what the hospital would have paid in taxes.

The Internal Revenue Service (IRS) articulated the idea of a "community benefit standard" to help judge hospitals' contributions in a 1969 ruling. In 2007, after almost 40 years of informal interpretation, the IRS added to Form 990 a Schedule H, which requires nonprofit hospitals to report various ways in which they contribute to the community they serve (IRS 2018). Compliance requirements were specified further in 2010 as part of the Affordable Care Act (ACA), and Schedule H was expanded accordingly.

Nonprofit hospitals wishing to maintain exemption from federal income tax must, among other tasks, define the community they serve, conduct a community health needs assessment every three years, identify other local organizations that respond to the community's needs, prepare a community health improvement plan, and be transparent with their community and patients about their financial aid policies. Activities pertaining to social determinants of health may be counted as community benefit contributions under certain circumstances, with detailed data provided.

Many of the cases in this book involve hospital initiatives related to the community. In some instances, the rationale for an activity is to fulfill the hospital's financial obligation to its community to maintain its tax-exempt status. But in other instances, the hospital becomes engaged with its community for other reasons, whether a sense of moral obligation, a desire to improve the overall well-being of the population, or a financial motive associated with the transition to value-based payment.

One excellent source of information about community benefit is the Catholic Health Association, an established leader in documenting healthcare organizations' contributions to their communities. The organization offers a variety of resources at www.chausa.org/communitybenefit/community-benefit.

Community Health Needs Assessment

A community health needs assessment (CHNA) has become a requirement for nonprofit community hospitals, Federally Qualified Health Centers, certain entities providing mental health services, Area Agencies on Aging, and sundry other organizations that receive funding from federal, state, or local government sources. Private accrediting agencies, such as the Public Health Accreditation Board, also require the organizations they accredit to conduct periodic needs assessments.

A comprehensive CHNA can involve all the elements of characterizing the community, identifying the components of the community health system, and mapping community assets, with all of these steps contributing toward a community health improvement plan aligned with the goals and mission of the leading organization.

Many communities had been conducting needs assessments prior to the release of the IRS CHNA requirements, but the types and quality of activities varied widely. Today, the CHNA requirements offer organizations an opportunity to do more than just meet minimum requirements; they offer a focus upon which to build collaborations with other organizations in the community, to become more data driven and evidence based, and to move beyond preparing reports to actually take actions that improve the health of the community (Deryk Van Brunt, Healthy Communities Institute, personal communication, 2018).

Case 3 describes the CHNA process in detail, examining how a health organization identifies potential health partner organizations in its community, compiles the essential primary and secondary data, and analyzes data to pinpoint the priorities of the community for subsequent interventions.

Community Health Improvement Plan

The term *community health improvement plan* (CHIP) can be broadly applied in a generic sense, or it can represent a specific, formal response by nonprofit hospitals to community benefit requirements. A CHIP serves as a guide to help organizations improve the health of the community's residents. A CHIP can be created in a variety of ways; no single process or template has been firmly established by the government or other sources. The IRS requires nonprofit hospitals to submit an implementation strategy but does not provide details about content or format.

Several cases in this book refer to a CHIP. Case 3, for instance, describes a process linking the CHNA and the CHIP for nonprofit hospitals in ways that meet IRS requirements. Case 6 asks the reader to be creative in developing a CHIP for a multiple-county collaborative.

References

County Health Rankings & Roadmaps. 2019. "How Healthy Is Your Community?" Accessed May 21. www.countyhealthrankings.org/.

French, J., and B. Raven. 1959. "The Bases of Social Power." In *Studies in Social Power*, edited by D. Cartwright, 150–67. Ann Arbor, MI: Institute for Social Research.

Internal Revenue Service (IRS). 2018. "2018 Instructions for Schedule H (Form 990)." Published November 20. www.irs.gov/pub/irs-pdf/i1040sh.pdf.

———. 1969. "Revenue Ruling 69-645, 1969-2, C.B. 117." Accessed May 22, 2019. www.irs.gov/pub/irs-tege/rr69-545.pdf.

McElroy, K. R., D. Bibeau, A. Steckler, and K. Glanz. 1988. "An Ecological Perspective on Health Promotion Programs." *Health Education Quarterly* 15 (4): 351–77.

US Department of Health and Human Services. 2019. "About Healthy People." Updated May 21. www.healthypeople.gov/2020/About-Healthy-People.

CHARACTERIZING A COMMUNITY: HEALTHFORALL HEALTH SYSTEM

Connie J. Evashwick

Case at a Glance

Overarching theme	The overarching theme of this case is to characterize the residents of a community, which includes defining the community and finding data about demographics, health behaviors, and health status.
Learning objectives	• Define a "community." • Describe a community according to the characteristics of its individuals and families. • Analyze a target audience for health status and the factors that affect health status. • Apply theories of health behavior to the health status of individuals and the community. • Compare the characteristics of a community and those of population subgroups. • Identify data sets relevant to the health status of a community. • Analyze trends in health status and health behaviors over time and in relationship to benchmarks. • Explain statistics of incidence, prevalence, rate, percentile, proportion, and index. • Define the management function of marketing, identify its key concepts, and explain its relevancy to characterizing a community.
Key terms	• Community • "Four Ps" of marketing • Managerial epidemiology • Marketing • Target audience
Management competency	Marketing
Population/subgroup	Community
Health issue or condition	Health status/behaviors

Management Challenge

HealthforAll Health System has purchased a hospital about which its leaders know very little. The purchase was part of a packaged deal, and HealthforAll does not know whether to keep the hospital, sell it, or close it altogether once the larger purchase is completed. HealthforAll's corporate office needs to acquire elementary but comprehensive data about the hospital, its operations, its financial status, and, perhaps most important of all, the community it serves.

Marketing can be defined as offering your target audience exactly the products they want, in the way they want them delivered, at the price they are willing to pay, and letting them know why your product is better than anyone else's. The key aspects of this definition reflect the "four Ps" of marketing: product, price, placement, and promotion. To succeed in marketing, an organization needs to understand its target audience and how its current and future products fit that audience's needs. This approach applies to services offered to communities and subpopulations, as well as to individuals.

HealthforAll needs to analyze the new hospital from a marketing perspective to determine whether the services, or "product," offered by the hospital have a viable future and how that future might be attained.

A Diagnostic Report

As part of a corporate purchase, HealthforAll Health System has purchased six hospitals in six different states. The system wanted four of the hospitals for flagship bases in large urban areas where they intended to gain a competitive edge. The other two hospitals were part of the deal, but HealthforAll did not know much about them. As a gesture of goodwill and to make a positive impression with the communities being served, HealthforAll intends to announce its presence by offering free vaccinations to anyone who has not received the immunizations recommended by the Centers for Disease Control and Prevention (CDC).

Maria Miller is the regional vice president for Hospital 5, one of the hospitals the HealthforAll corporate office knows little about. The HealthforAll office has asked her to provide a complete diagnostic report about the hospital, in three parts: Part 1 is to describe the status of internal operations and finances at the hospital; part 2 is to focus on the community served by the hospital and assess the potential for a revised set of services; and part 3 is to provide an estimate of how much vaccine of various types would be needed to bring the community to full immunization status.

Maria is comfortable doing part 1 of the report, given that she has spent 30 years with the hospital, first as a nurse and then as a hospital administrator. Part 2, however, seems more daunting. For part 2, important data would include the following:

- The community
  - Demographics (e.g., age, gender, family status)
  - Education
  - Employment
  - Income
  - Languages
  - Ethnicities/culture
  - Religion
- Health status
  - Morbidity and major causes of hospitalization
  - Mortality—major causes
  - Maternal mortality
  - Infant mortality
  - Births, teen births
  - Mental health indicators
  - Other notable key health indicators
- Health behaviors
  - Smoking
  - Obesity
  - Sexually transmitted diseases
  - Binge drinking
  - Alcohol abuse
  - Opioid use or drug overdose
  - Teenage pregnancy

The Science of Epidemiology

The *Farlex Partner Medical Dictionary* (2012) defines *epidemiology* is as "the study of the distribution and determinants of health-related states or events in specified populations, and the application of this study to control of health problems." The English doctor John Snow is regarded as the father of modern epidemiology. During an epidemic of cholera in London in 1854, Snow noticed that cases were located near the Broad Street water pump, and he convinced community leaders to remove the handle of the pump, stopping the flow of contaminated water to the community. The epidemic soon ended. Managerial epidemiology is the application of epidemiology principles to the management and operations of health services.

- Healthcare utilization
  - Hospital inpatient care
  - Hospital outpatient care
  - Physician utilization
  - Health insurance coverage

Part 3 should be straightforward once the characteristics of the population are known. Relevant data on immunizations would include the following:

- CDC guidelines, by population subgroup
- State average immunization rates
- Local immunization rates

Maria engages an intern from the nearby university's school of public health, and she asks the intern to identify the information needed for part 2 of the report. She also asks the intern to determine what data are readily available through secondary data sources and what data will require primary data collection. Finally, she asks the intern to outline the information and the calculations that would be needed for part 3.

Personal Perspective

Julia, age 39, and her family had come from Latin America to the United States to seek asylum. Accompanying her were her 60-year-old mother, her 15-year-old daughter, her 12-year-old son, and her 2-year-old daughter. All speak Spanish but not English. Julia and her family members had lacked access to any regular healthcare in their native country. Upon arrival in the United States, she went to a community health center that welcomes immigrants, and the doctor recommended that she and all her family members receive routine immunizations appropriate for their ages. The children are required to have full immunizations before they can attend public schools, and Julia and her mother want to get the proper immunizations so that they will remain healthy. However, the family has no money to pay for care. They have heard that the local hospital might be offering free immunizations in the near future.

Questions

Fact and Data Analysis Questions

1. How will Hospital 5 define its "community"? What alternative definitions might it consider?

2. What is the difference between secondary and primary data?

3. Describe five ways to collect primary data. What are the benefits and limits of each method?

4. Describe five ways to collect secondary data. What are the benefits and limits of each method?

5. How are geographic areas relevant to data about populations and communities?

6. What is the single most consistent data set compiled for the US population? How frequently are the data collected?

7. Find and critique six data sets that contain demographic data pertaining to a community you define.

8. Find six data sets that have information pertaining to healthcare status, healthcare services utilization, and healthcare behaviors.

9. What is epidemiology?

10. Define *incidence*, *prevalence*, *rate*, *ratio*, *percent*, *proportion*, and *index*.

11. Define *marketing*.

12. What are the "four Ps" of marketing?

13. Describe four theories of health behavior.

Discussion Questions

1. Contrast the definitions of *community*, *population*, and *target audience*. How can the size of each be measured?

2. In applying or comparing data from secondary data sets, describe the key considerations relating to the following:
   - Definitions
   - Measures
   - Metrics
   - Date of data collection
   - Sample selection criteria

3. What are the benefits and drawbacks of using a single data set, such as the County Health Rankings, as the major source of data to describe the health needs of the community?

4. What data does the Centers for Disease Control and Prevention website offer pertaining to the health of a community?

5. How do theories of health behavior pertain to the health of a community?

6. Describe the key issues in relating data about inpatients and utilization to data about the community.

7. What would HealthforAll Health System want to know about the community and population groups served by Hospital 5 that is not readily available in existing data sets (i.e., available secondary data)? What methods could be used to

gather that information (i.e., collect primary data)? Identify the essential missing information and cost-effective ways of gathering it in a three-month time frame.

8. Compare data for the hospital's community to benchmarks for the state and for the nation. How can such comparisons contribute to decision making about the hospital's current and future programs?

9. Assume the hospital proceeds with its outreach effort to offer free immunizations to anyone in the community who has not had the vaccinations recommended by the CDC. Although this program seems like a positive initiative, what challenges might it face? What are realistic targets for success? In addition to the CDC, what other sources recommend or endorse vaccinations? Are all sources consistent in their recommendations?

10. From a healthcare institution's perspective, how can the functions and concepts of marketing be applied to characterizing its community as well as its patients?

Reference

Farlex Partner Medical Dictionary. 2012. "Epidemiology." Accessed May 22, 2019. https://medical-dictionary.thefreedictionary.com/epidemiology.

Useful Resources

Websites

- American Community Survey (www.census.gov/programs-surveys/acs/)
- Behavioral Risk Factor Surveillance Survey System (www.cdc.gov/brfss/index.html)
- Centers for Disease Control and Prevention (www.cdc.gov)
- CDC Community Health Improvement Navigator (www.cdc.gov/chinav/)
- CDC Tools for Social Determinants of Health (www.cdc.gov/socialdeterminants/)
- Community Toolbox (https://ctb.ku.edu/en)
- Substance Abuse and Mental Health Services Administration (www.samhsa.gov)
- US Census Bureau (www.census.gov)

Books

- *Essentials of Health Behavior*, 3rd ed. (Jones & Bartlett, 2020), by Mark Edberg
- *Marketing Health Services*, 3rd ed. (Health Administration Press, 2014), by Richard K. Thomas
- *Marketing Tools for Healthcare Executives* (Oxford Crest, 2020), by John L. Fortenberry Jr.

2

COMMUNITY ASSET MAPPING: SHARP HEALTHCARE SENIOR HEALTH CENTER

Jillian Warriner

Note: This case is generally based on the structure and attributes of Sharp HealthCare, but changes have been made and details added for pedagogical purposes.

Case at a Glance

Overarching theme	The focus of this chapter is community asset mapping.
Learning objectives	• Analyze a target community for demographic and economic characteristics. • Describe the need for seniors with complex chronic illnesses to have access within their community to a comprehensive set of services. • Define a continuum of care for seniors. • Identify the assets in a community. • Evaluate community assets with a focus on finding potential partners to provide a continuum of care to seniors. • Assess the dynamics of power among agencies within a community. • Develop the interorganizational relationships required to give seniors access to a comprehensive continuum of care. • Identify the business model by which a health organization can create a continuum of care through partnership arrangements.
Key terms	• Activities of daily living (ADLs) • Caregiving • Chronic condition • Community asset • Community asset mapping • Community-based organizations (CBOs) • Continuum of care • Formal power

- For-profit organization
- Geriatrics
- Gerontology
- Goals and objectives
- Informal power
- Instrumental activities of daily living (IADLs)
- Medicaid
- Medicare
- Mission
- Nonprofit/not-for-profit organization
- Social determinants of health (SDoH)
- Sources of power
- Supplemental insurance
- Values
- Vision

Management competencies	Marketing, strategic planning, business plan development
Population/ subgroups	Seniors, health professions workforce, caregivers
Health issue or condition	Multifaceted conditions, chronic conditions of seniors (including functional abilities)

Management Challenge

Sharp HealthCare (Sharp) is one of the dominant health systems serving the county of San Diego, California. The only major health system that focuses specifically on senior health, it has two Senior Health Centers (SHCs) and two Senior Resource Centers. As the aging population of San Diego County grows, Sharp is considering adding a third SHC to serve the community. This decision would be consistent with the findings of its recent community health needs assessment (Sharp HealthCare 2019). The challenge is to determine where the center should be located and what specific programs and services it should offer.

Sharp recognizes the importance of providing a continuum of care for seniors, with some services offered directly, some through formal partners, and some through informal referrals. Sharp must identify appropriate community partners to build this continuum for seniors as well as their caregivers. Thus, identifying and evaluating specific community assets are critical components of the program proposal. The staff have begun to gather an array of data to determine the location, service package, and community partners appropriate for the new SHC.

Background

Sharp HealthCare was first established in 1955 as Donald N. Sharp Memorial Community Hospital. Since that time, Sharp has expanded to serve San Diego County with four acute care hospitals, three specialty hospitals, three affiliated medical groups, a commercial health plan (Sharp Health Plan), and more than 18,000 employees. Sharp Health Plan provides individual and family plans, employer-sponsored group plans, and Medicare plans, including a Medicare Advantage plan. Further, Sharp is also a leading provider of care to the Medi-Cal (Medicaid) population in San Diego County, and Sharp Health Plan provides coverage options through Covered California (California's state Medicaid program). A map of San Diego County, with Sharp facility locations, is shown in exhibit 2.1.

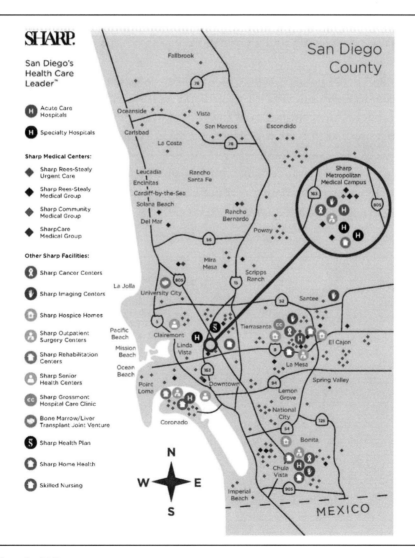

EXHIBIT 2.1

Map of San Diego with Location of Sharp Hospitals and Senior Health Centers

Source: Sharp HealthCare.

Currently, Sharp operates two Senior Health Centers and two Senior Resource Centers. The SHCs offer clinical services from geriatricians and geriatric nurse practitioners, as well as an array of other services tailored specifically for seniors. Sharp's SHCs help coordinate the following services:

- Billing for Medicare and supplemental insurance
- Health education programs and community resources
- Home health care referrals and coordination
- Health screenings
- Insurance billing and assistance
- Medication management
- Primary physician care with 24-hour emergency coverage
- Podiatry
- Specialty care referrals and coordination

Each of the SHCs has arrangements, either formal or informal, with local community providers who offer health-related and social services. Sharp has used a long-standing model of the continuum of care (Evashwick 1987) to identify and organize these services so that the care is efficient and effective for seniors with complex, multifaceted needs (see exhibit 2.2).

Sharp's Senior Resource Centers are on-site departments at two of its acute care hospitals. They engage primarily in education, outreach, screening, and support for senior patients and community members; they do not offer clinical services.

EXHIBIT 2.2
Continuum of
Care Model

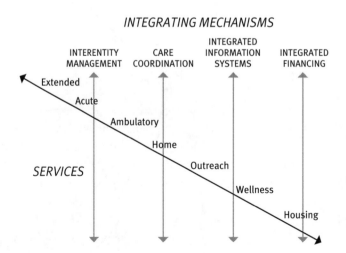

Source: Evashwick (1987).

In evaluating the options for a new SHC, Sharp must answer the following questions:

- Where in San Diego County should the center be located, based on current and projected demographics?
- What services should Sharp offer directly on site?
- What services should Sharp offer through collaboration with community partners?

Further, in preparing the business case for a new SHC, Sharp must clarify for both its finance committee and the board of directors the rationale for a distinct program based on the unique needs of seniors.

Needs of Seniors

The rationale for creating a separate clinic for seniors is the fact that people aged 65 or older require care unique to their age demographic. The physical and mental health challenges of aging are well documented, and seniors often have multiple, complex, chronic health conditions that complicate optimum care and medication management.

Another critical component of the health and well-being of seniors is socialization. Seniors who lack a caregiver at home or who are otherwise socially isolated face increased fall risk, greater behavioral health risks, and more significant cognitive decline, as well as challenges with transportation to both medical appointments and other critical resources (e.g., food). Moreover, many seniors face daily challenges performing activities of daily living (e.g., eating, bathing, dressing) or instrumental activities of daily living (e.g., housework, transportation, management of finances), and quality of life becomes a significant issue.

Personal Perspective

Helena is a 98-year-old widow who lives in her home of 60 years. She has been diagnosed as profoundly deaf, with some degree of dementia and unsteady balance. She has been a frequent visitor to the emergency room because of repeated falls. After her most recent visit to the hospital, she was admitted to a skilled nursing facility for rehabilitation. After two months, she is returning home with a long list of recommendations:

- For the next six weeks, participate in physical therapy twice a week.
- Get a walker.

(continued)

- Upgrade her hearing aid.
- Use a remote-control Bluetooth device to control the volume on the television.
- Change the bathtub in the downstairs bathroom to a shower.
- Arrange for a cleaning person to come in once a week.
- Sign up for Meals on Wheels and request lunches Monday through Friday.
- Engage a home care agency to send a home health aide for four hours three times a week.
- Sign up for Dial-A-Lift to arrange for transportation to physical therapy and doctor appointments.
- Have prescriptions put on automatic renewal and home delivery.
- Sign up for a free program to obtain a telephone with volume and text control.
- Find a new doctor and enroll in the doctor's panel.
- Switch her Medicare plan at the next open enrollment cycle.

Helena's family wonders how they are going to get the services set up, let alone maintain them over time.

Continuum of Care

A *continuum of care* can be defined as "an integrated, client-oriented system of care composed of both services and integrating mechanisms that guides and tracks clients over time through a comprehensive array of health, mental health, and social services spanning all levels of intensity of care" (Evashwick 1987, 23).

An array of services is necessary to meet the multiple needs of older adults. Seniors might spend five days in a hospital, but for the remaining 360 days of the year they receive care at home and tap into community resources. In considering a new SHC, Sharp must determine what additional age-related services are important to its patients, as well as which community-based organizations (CBOs) offer those services. Moreover, in light of the various payment programs that Sharp offers seniors, the following points must be taken into account when considering the new center's financial viability:

- What resources for seniors already exist in the community?
- What services should Sharp offer directly, and which would be offered through informal or formal referrals to other agencies serving the community?
- How should partner agencies be selected?

- How should partnerships be managed for financial efficiency and patient quality? With which agencies should Sharp seek to arrange formal partnerships? Which agencies should remain informal partners?
- What measures will be used to assess the success of the center?
- What elements will be essential to include in a formal communications plan to the community, so that the new SHC attracts clients immediately?

Asset Mapping

The likely geographic location for Sharp's next SHC is "South County," or the area in the southern end of San Diego County. To assess potential partners for either formal or informal relationships, Sharp must first identify the agencies that are already serving seniors in this general area. In addition, Sharp considers agencies that are based in other parts of San Diego County but that could potentially expand to collaborate with the new SHC if the volume and funding were sufficient to attract their investment. Sharp embarks on asset mapping using several steps:

1. *Mapping the service area.* Sharp uses internal hospital discharge data to map its service area—that is, the communities (often at the zip code level) where its patients reside and the types of services most commonly used after discharge (see exhibits 2.3 and 2.4).

Discharge Disposition	Age 64–74	Age 75–84	Age 85+	Total
Home/self-care (routine)	55.89%	44.24%	29.24%	44.79%
Skilled nursing	17.44%	24.22%	31.63%	23.53%
Home health service	14.96%	18.84%	21.29%	17.94%
All other	6.55%	8.00%	12.56%	8.69%
Short-term acute	2.25%	2.12%	1.98%	2.13%
Board/care residential	0.74%	0.40%	0.37%	0.53%
Rehab	0.69%	0.74%	0.66%	0.70%
Long-term acute	0.62%	0.64%	0.32%	0.54%
Psych. hospital	0.49%	0.20%	0.06%	0.28%
Assisted living	0.37%	0.60%	1.89%	0.87%

EXHIBIT 2.3
Sharp Hospital Discharge Dispositions for Patients Aged 64 or Older, 2017

Source: Sharp HealthCare internal databases, 2017.

EXHIBIT 2.4
Mapping of
Discharges

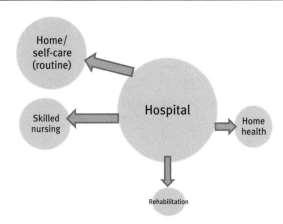

Note: Size of bubble indicates magnitude.

2. *Identifying potential partners.* The types of agencies/partners sought are based on the Continuum of Care Model. Sharp's planning staff embark on the process of finding out what resources and programs serve the designated geographic area. Sharp begins by asking hospital staff—including social workers, case managers, and discharge planners—which agencies currently serve as collaborators to address patients' needs upon discharge. Sharp may also check with 211 San Diego, the San Diego Department of Health and Human Services office serving that region, Aging and Independence Services, and other current partners to obtain contact information for new CBOs with which it might collaborate. Sharp conducts key informant interviews with nurses or administrators of physician practices in the area, and it contacts local churches to ask what social support services might be available. Sharp's planners also meet with representatives from the county's Department of Transportation to learn about public transportation routes, dial-a-ride programs, and local proprietary agencies, ranging from taxis to ride-sharing companies.

3. *Evaluating partners.* Armed with a list of potential community assets, Sharp's planning staff begin the process of evaluating each of the potential partners for quality indicators, reputation, financial stability, service area, and capacity of staff to provide services, as well as power within the community. Sharp uses a table, shown in exhibit 2.5, to facilitate easy comparison. For most services within the continuum of care for seniors, accreditation or licensing bodies provide information and metrics on select criteria. However, each service has distinct accreditation or quality measures, so a separate assessment is done for quality (see exhibit 2.6). In addition, potential partners must meet criteria for risk and financial performance.

4. *Assessing power.* Power, both formal and informal, is an intangible characteristic, but it is incorporated into the analysis as well.

EXHIBIT 2.5
Organizational Partnership Assessment

Organization	Mission	Services	Clients	Geography (region served)	Payment sources	Cost/ service	Can these services be provided internally (via Sharp)?	Length of time CBO has been in the community	Does the CBO work with other health systems?
A									
B									
C									
D									
E									
F									
G									
H									
I									

EXHIBIT 2.6
Organizational
Partnership
Assessment for
Quality

Service	Accreditation Body	Quality Sites	Measures of Quality
A			
B			

Note: List continues for all letters in previous exhibit.

Sharp must project the approximate demand for each service based on the total client pool expected at the SHC, as well as the health and social conditions likely to be observed. The selection of CBO partners must have the capacity to meet the needs of the projected patient volume. For example, a small home health agency might offer high quality but be limited in total capacity. Sharp must then decide if contracts with two agencies/CBOs would be essential or if one contract with a larger agency would be simpler, assuming the quality would be closely monitored. Additionally, the CBOs must have their own incentives to participate in a collaborative effort with Sharp.

Caregivers and Workforce

Sharp's SHCs are a resource for more than just senior patients. Families, informal and formal caregivers, and health professionals are all affected by the services they provide.

The act of caregiving is closely tied to the health and protection of seniors, and research shows that caregivers often endure a high degree of stress. Formal caregivers are often paid low wages, and informal caregivers often serve as a hidden workforce, conducting extremely challenging and time-consuming work out of a sense of family duty. In addition, many nonfamily caregivers are compensated privately (without regulation), and thus their numbers are not accurately represented in workforce statistics.

In San Diego, the matching of caregivers with seniors in need is particularly complex. The area's demographics reveal numerous ethnic groups with a variety of cultures, including 18 tribes of American Indians; a strong military presence, with many military families coming and going; and countless languages, ranging from Spanish to Somali.

Providing care for seniors also requires a full array of health professionals. Seniors often need both acute and ongoing care for multiple, often co-occurring, chronic health conditions (e.g., heart disease, diabetes), as well as behavioral health support and social support. To facilitate coordination among the various professionals, case managers (also known as care coordinators) may become involved at the request of insurance plans, service systems, or families.

Financial Arrangements

The new SHC is expected to be a positive business line for Sharp HealthCare. Currently, Sharp's SHCs serve the following primary payer categories: Medicare contracts, Medicare Advantage contracts, dual Medicare/Medicaid contracts (known as "Medi-Medis"), other government contracts, self-pay by individuals and families, and private payers, either HMO or PPO.

The proportion of payments for Sharp's two existing SHCs is shown in exhibit 2.7. The new center is expected to be financed primarily through managed care health plans, including Medicare, Medicare Advantage, Medi-Cal (Medicaid), and other government programs. The financial composition is anticipated to be in relation to the demographics of the area. Sharp's project planning staff will remind Sharp's board of directors and finance committee of the various payment methods by providing a summary chart of coverage by payment type.

In addition to the incentives associated with payment through Medicare Advantage, Sharp has a financial interest in the continuum of care as a way to reduce avoidable costs. For instance, significant cost savings can be achieved when CBO programs and support serve as a supplement to patients' medical care, helping to meet the social service needs of patients after discharge from the hospital. Such services not only can help patients avoid inpatient readmissions and emergency room visits; they can also

EXHIBIT 2.7
Payment Arrangements for Sharp's Existing Senior Health Centers

Sharp Senior Health Center: Clairemont

Category	Pct.
Medicare (traditional)	88.14%
Medicare Advantage	6.76%
Dual Medicare & Medi-Cal	4.90%
Other government	0.11%
HMO	0.05%
Self-pay	0.03%
PPO	0.02%

Sharp Senior Health Center: Downtown

Category	Pct.
Medicare (traditional)	36.89%*
Dual Medicare & Medi-Cal	49.12%
Medicare Advantage	12.88%
Self-pay	1.04%
PPO	0.07%

*In 2017, nearly 18% of this category was aligned with Sharp HealthCare's NextGen ACO.
Source: Data from Sharp Healthcare internal databases, 2017.

enable seniors to thrive in the management of their health outside the hospital walls, thus greatly improving quality of life.

Sharp's SHC team has compiled a wealth of data related to the location, services, partners, and expected financial performance of the new center, but decisions about each of these areas remain to be made. The staff submit their report and recommendations to the leadership team of Sharp HealthCare and await the results.

Questions

Fact and Data Analysis Questions

1. What is the definition of a "senior"? What is the significance of age 65?
2. What do demographic trends say about the senior population?
3. Compare the frequency and costs of healthcare utilization by seniors with the frequency and costs of utilization by younger adults.
4. What is asset mapping?
5. What are the bases for power? For one perspective, see French and Raven (1959).
6. What is the official definition of a "chronic condition"? What are ADLs? IADLs?
7. What is Medicare? What services of the continuum of care does it cover? Who is eligible?
8. What is Medicaid? What services of the continuum of care does it cover? Who is eligible?
9. What is a continuum of care? Why is it relevant to services for seniors?
10. Who are caregivers? Why are they relevant to a continuum of care for seniors?

Discussion Questions

1. How does an organization find the assets in its community that are relevant to its business?
2. Describe the types of health, mental health, and social services available for seniors in a typical community.
3. How does a person's functional status, as measured by ADLs and IADLs, relate to the need for a continuum of care?
4. Are members of the health professions workforce considered assets in a community? How are they counted?

5. What does the Internal Revenue Service Form 990, Schedule H, require of not-for-profit hospitals in reporting community assets? Why must assets be reported?

6. Describe the links that exist among services in a community provided to a single individual.

7. What is 211? Does your community have such a system? Why has 211 developed separately from the healthcare system?

8. How many organizations should Sharp identify as potential partners for its Senior Health Center? Which ones should be the highest priority? What criteria should they use to decide?

9. If the members of the Sharp C-suite attend a chamber of commerce meeting and announce their new Senior Health Center and partners, what reactions can they expect from other organizational leaders? How will they explain their selection process and criteria?

10. How can the power of organizations in a community be evaluated and compared?

11. Once Sharp decides on its partners for the SHC, how will the relationships be structured? Will contracts or memoranda of understanding be used? What will be the financial arrangements? How will services be coordinated from a management perspective, as well as from a client perspective?

12. What approach would Sharp take if it discovers that the home health agency that best meets its criteria for a partner home care provider already partners with one of the competing health systems in San Diego?

13. Once Sharp establishes relationships with partners and starts operation of its new SHC, what criteria and methods will it use to evaluate the success of those partnerships?

14. What happens if expected organizational partnerships do not work out? What might be reasons for the relationships not to succeed?

15. Should asset mapping be a confidential process, kept within the purview of the C-suite, board, and program directors?

References

Evashwick, C. 1987. "Definition of the Continuum of Care." In *Managing the Continuum of Care*, edited by C. Evashwick and L. Weiss, 23–44. Rockville, MD: Aspen Publishers.

French, J., and B. Raven. 1959. "The Bases of Social Power." In *Studies in Social Power*, edited by D. Cartwright, 150–67. Ann Arbor, MI: Institute for Social Research.

Sharp HealthCare. 2019. "Community Health Needs Assessments." Accessed May 30. www.sharp.com/about/community/community-benefits/health-needs-assessments.cfm.

Useful Resources

- Older Americans Act (https://acl.gov/about-acl/older-americans-act-oaa)
- US Department of Health and Human Services—Aging (www.hhs.gov/aging)
- US Department of Health and Human Services—Programs for Seniors (www.hhs.gov/programs/social-services/programs-for-seniors/index.html)
- "What Is Asset Mapping?" by AmeriCorps VISTA Campus (www.vistacampus.gov/what-asset-mapping)

CONDUCTING A COMMUNITY HEALTH NEEDS ASSESSMENT

Deryk Van Brunt, Claire Lindsay, Sheila Baxter, Kimberly Peeren, Andrew Juhnke, Sophia Blachman-Biatch, and Jenny Belforte

Note: Some content in this chapter has been adapted from Conduent Healthy Communities Institute's Community Health Needs Assessment Guide (see www.conduent.com/ community-population-health/community-health-assessment/).

Case at a Glance

Overarching theme	The focus of this case is the process for conducting a community health needs assessment.
Learning objectives	• Explain the purpose of performing a community health needs assessment (CHNA). • Delineate the main steps in performing a CHNA. • Critique data, data collection methods, and data presentation techniques. • Prioritize community health needs.
Key terms	• Community benefit • Community health needs assessment (CHNA) • Disparity • Primary data • Prioritization • Reliability • Secondary data • Social determinants of health (SDoH) • Validity
Management competencies	Project planning, marketing, informatics
Population/subgroup	Many options
Health issue or condition	Any

Management Challenge

Oak Grove Hospital faces a major task for the coming fiscal year: conducting its community health needs assessment (CNHA). Not-for-profit hospitals in the United States are required by the Internal Revenue Service (IRS) to demonstrate their benefit to the community by performing a CHNA once every three years. The hospitals must then develop an implementation strategy (IS) to address community health needs that the CHNA identified as significant (Health Services Research Information Central 2019). The hospitals must report their activities to the IRS annually on Form 990, Schedule H. A snapshot of CHNA requirements is shown in exhibit 3.1.

The basic logic behind this requirement is that, if nonprofit hospitals are exempt from paying taxes because they provide an essential benefit to the community, they should have a thorough understanding of the community's health needs so that they can target resources and develop plans to address those needs. In addition to their mandated use by nonprofit hospitals, CHNAs can also help organizations of various types to collaborate and collectively become more data driven and evidence based in their approach to improving community health.

Oak Grove Hospital's leaders need to make four key decisions before delegating the assessment process to the director of the Community Benefit Department.

- What research methods are best for the CHNA and the subsequent IS? What data are available from secondary sources? What must be gathered through primary data collection?
- Which, if any, other organization(s) should they partner with to conduct the CHNA?

EXHIBIT 3.1
Snapshot of
IRS Community
Health Needs
Assessment
Requirements

- Define the **service area.**
- Describe the service area's **demographics.**
- **Analyze health data** to identify health needs in the community and identifiable disparities.
- Gather **community input**, especially from public health experts and vulnerable populations.
- Determine **significant health needs** by considering findings from the data analysis and community input.
- **Identify resources** available to meet the identified significant health needs.
- **Prioritize** the significant health needs in the community, with community input.
- **Evaluate** the impact of any actions that were taken in the three years since the last CHNA was completed.
- **Adopt the CHNA** formally, by board approval or equivalent.
- **Share the CHNA report** with the community for public comment.

Note: These components were specified in 2014 as a result of the terms articulated in the Affordable Care Act of 2010. This information is subject to change; check the IRS website for current requirements.

Source: IRS (2014).

- How should they prioritize needs once the data have been collected?
- What resources must the hospital allocate for the CHNA?

Background: Oak Grove Community Hospital

Oak Grove Community Hospital is a 350-bed nonprofit hospital serving the counties of Franklin and Oso. In total, three hospitals serve the region: Oak Grove Community Hospital; one smaller not-for-profit hospital in Oso County, which collaborates with Oak Grove on an annual health fair using English-Spanish materials and activities; and one midsized for-profit hospital with a similar service area to Oak Grove's and a historically competitive relationship. In addition to these hospitals, a range of community-based organizations—including local schools, the United Way, the regional YMCA, and faith-based organizations—are involved in service and health improvement activities.

In the past, the two not-for-profit hospitals have completed their CHNAs individually, while the third hospital has done a private "community analysis." This year, however, Pat Mendoza, the CEO of the smaller not-for-profit hospital, proposed that the three hospitals collaborate, given their overlapping service areas and their desire to be more efficient with personnel and resources.

Cathy White, the CEO of Oak Grove, weighed the pros and cons of collaborating on the CHNA. She considered suggesting to her board that Oak Grove not only collaborate with the other hospitals but also work with the local public health department, the Federally Qualified Health Center, the nearby mental health clinic, and even the Area Agency on Aging—all of which are required to conduct periodic needs assessments if they are to receive federal money.

Ultimately, Frank Matsu, the CEO of the for-profit hospital, convinced Cathy that collaboration among the three hospitals was a good approach for this round. Frank felt that the hospitals could effect greater change in the community by working together. They could always add more participants in the future—assuming the initial relationship went smoothly.

As a first step, the three hospitals established the Oak Grove CHNA Task Force. Community health representatives from each hospital's staff were put in charge of spearheading efforts and bringing a plan back to their organization's senior management. They recognized that each of the organizations had slightly different reasons and thus goals for participating in the collaborative CHNA effort.

The Community Health Needs Assessment Process

The Task Force proposed a six-step process for conducting the CHNA, as shown in exhibit 3.2.

EXHIBIT 3.2
Steps in the
Community
Health Needs
Assessment
Process

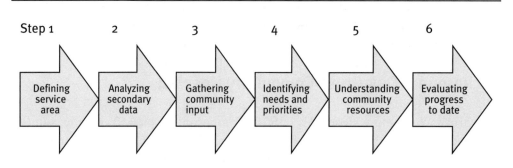

Step 1: Define the Service Area

The first step is to define the service area of the hospital or organization spearheading the CHNA. The service area can be defined using standard geographic units of the counties, cities, zip codes, or census tracts being served. Service areas may also include specialized geographies, such as metropolitan statistical areas, multiple-county regions, neighborhoods, and election districts.

Additionally, a service area can be defined by a specialized target population, such as children, women, people with disabilities, or the elderly. For example, the service area for a children's hospital would focus specifically on the subpopulation of children in the defined geographic area.

Per IRS regulations, a hospital facility may not define its service area to exclude medically underserved, low-income, or minority populations living in the geographic area from which the facility draws its patients. A hospital facility must take into account all patients in the service area without regard to whether, or how much, they or their insurers pay for care received.

A justification should be provided for the organization's selected and defined service area. For example, a given county might be chosen as a hospital's service area because a substantial percentage of the hospital's patient population resides in that county.

The Oak Grove CNHA Task Force defined its service area as the counties of Franklin and Oso, as well as all the cities, census places, zip codes, and census tracts therein. Nearly 100 percent of the three hospitals' patient population resides in one of those two counties.

Franklin County contains 13 cities and an additional 25 census-designated places, with a total population of 405,890. Oso County contains 6 cities and an additional 15 census-designated places, for a total population of 228,172. The entire hospital service area, therefore, includes 634,062 people.

The smaller not-for-profit hospital serves patients and offers community activities primarily in Franklin County. Pat Mendoza, the CEO, agreed to use the larger service area as long as key data could be broken down by individual county rather than aggregated. Everyone realized that organizing the data in this manner would take a bit more staff time, but the incremental cost was worthwhile to keep the hospital from dropping out of the collaborative effort.

Leaders of the black and Hispanic/Latino communities in the two counties suspect that major disparities in health status affect members of those groups. The Task Force representatives, therefore, proposed to their respective organizations that the CHNA take these subpopulations into special account. The Task Force does not want critical subgroups of the community to feel that they are underrepresented or that their needs are not adequately documented in the CHNA.

Step 2: Analyze Available (Secondary) Data

The initial phase of data analysis focuses on finding and examining three distinct types of data: demographic data, health data, and societal and environmental data. Data that have already been collected by an independent third-party entity and put into a database available for analysis are known as *secondary data*. A list of strengths and weaknesses of secondary data is provided in exhibit 3.3.

Demographic Data

The Oak Grove Task Force was aware that demographic data were readily available from a variety of sources, including the US Census and the American Community Survey. Analysis of that demographic data would examine age, race/ethnicity, gender, education, income, poverty, language, and disability status. Measures can be presented as numbers, percentages, ranges, or ratios and compared to a benchmark or standard. Demographic data might also include such figures as how many people speak a language other than English at home, how many are high school graduates, what percentage have

Strengths	Weaknesses
Data are replicable.	Data can lag; periods of measure are often more than a year.
Data have been validated.	Data collection methodologies may differ across sources.
Data are often publicly available for free.	Data from different sources may not be comparable to one another.
Many types of different data are available.	The purpose for which the data were collected may differ from yours, thus questions might not be asked in precisely the way you would like for your purpose.
Data sets are relatively easy to obtain at any time.	Data sources may not consistently update the data, so that data might be old.

EXHIBIT 3.3
Strengths and Weaknesses of Secondary Data

attained a bachelor's degree, the median household income, and the ratio of persons living below the poverty level to those above the poverty level.

In using data from secondary sources, the Task Force had to evaluate data for their availability, validity, and reliability. Then, the data had to be reported and displayed using metrics that can be easily understood by the audience.

Data for the two-county service area defined by the Oak Grove CHNA Task Force revealed the following:

- Population measures such as overall growth rate, age trends, and trends in race/ethnicity show a population that is increasingly diverse.
- Several zip codes indicate a high percentage of people who speak a language other than English at home.
- Education disparities are seen between the communities having higher percentages of black and Hispanic/Latino residents and the communities having a higher percentage of white residents.
- Data on income, poverty, and unemployment levels by zip code show variation in socioeconomic status, with two zip codes in Oso County showing particularly low levels on all three variables.

Creating Meaningful Measures

Data on socioeconomic factors can be combined to measure the overall effect of these various elements on the health status of the community. The SocioNeeds Index, developed by the Conduent Healthy Communities Institute, and the ratings from County Health Rankings are two examples of indexes used to score and rank geographic areas (such as counties or zip codes) within a service area by how much socioeconomic need they have.

The SocioNeeds Index incorporates estimates for six different social and economic determinants of health—income, poverty, unemployment, occupation, education attainment, and linguistic barriers—that are associated with premature death and preventable causes of hospitalization (Conduent Healthy Communities Institute 2018). Social and economic factors are well known to be strong determinants of health outcomes, with people of low socioeconomic status being more likely to be affected by chronic conditions such as diabetes, obesity, and cancer. Thus, socioeconomic analysis can help organizations focus on communities that can benefit most from targeted programs or policies.

Health Data

To find information about the health status of the residents of its service area, the Oak Grove Task Force started with an analysis of secondary data. The members focused on three types of sources:

- The Task Force reviewed data from national sources, including the American Community Survey, the National Cancer Institute, the Centers for Disease

Control and Prevention, the Environmental Protection Agency, the County Health Rankings, and the American Lung Association (see exhibit 3.4).

- The Task Force reviewed data from state sources, including the state Department of Education, the state Department of Public Health, the state Department of Justice, the state's School Kids Survey, and the state's Health Interview Survey.

- The Task Force reviewed previously collected data from a survey administered in the community by some of Oak Grove's partners (the YMCA in conjunction with the United Way and the counties' school districts). The survey measured residents' attitudes on health, health status, and health behaviors. When possible, the Task Force compared the data to local targets, because all city governments in Franklin County delineated guidelines for health progress, which included targets for statuses and behaviors to be met by 2021.

For the secondary data analysis, a clear method must be established for how community needs will be identified from the results, to standardize the analysis and to make the assessment replicable. The analysis should systematically look at how data points for a geography of interest perform against other geographies. For example, for a given indicator or measurement, the data value for a county can be compared to the data value for the state within which the county falls. Alternatively, county data values can be compared to data values for other counties within the same state.

In addition to helping identify topic areas of need, secondary data analysis can reveal subpopulation disparities, which are crucial to understanding health in the community. Subpopulation disparities may exist by age, race/ethnicity, gender, education level, or income level, and they can be identified in a variety of ways—including by comparing data value confidence intervals for each subpopulation subcategory to the overall data value confidence intervals. Disparities can be identified by indicator and can also be summarized across health or quality-of-life topic areas.

- American Community Survey
- American Lung Association
- Behavioral Risk Factor Surveillance System
- Centers for Disease Control and Prevention
- Centers for Medicare & Medicaid Services
- County Health Rankings
- Feeding America
- National Cancer Institute
- National Center for Education Statistics
- Small Area Health Insurance Estimates
- US Department of Agriculture's Food Environment Atlas
- US Environmental Protection Agency
- Youth Risk Behavior Surveillance System

EXHIBIT 3.4
Sources of Available Data on Health Issues

Oak Grove's secondary data analysis of health data revealed the following issues:

- Exercise, nutrition, and weight are a priority problem in the region, with adolescents and Hispanic/Latino community members faring worse than the community overall.
- Other health-related issue areas included access to health services, transportation, heart disease and stroke, substance abuse, and cancer.
- In both Franklin and Oso counties, the rates for obesity/overweight are better than the overall state value, but an upward (harmful) trend has appeared over the past four measurement periods.

Zip code–level analysis revealed that two zip codes in Franklin County and one zip code in Oso County have especially significant need in the areas of exercise, nutrition, and weight; heart disease; and substance abuse.

Societal and Environmental Data

Using the Ecological Model of Health (which illustrates that health is shaped by different spheres of influence, including policy and environmental factors), the Oak Grove Task Force sought to consider all factors in the greater environment that might lead to local health needs. The members decided to focus on access to health services and transportation as two key elements that they knew were frequent problems for the people of the two counties. Using recent state and local reports, they found data about the prevalence of health insurance, enrollment in the state's Medicaid program, and two measures of transportation reported by local authorities.

Step 3: Gather Community Input (Primary Data)

Whereas secondary data analysis begins the process of identifying key areas of need for the community assessment, community input integrates immediate and direct community ideas and opinions. Data gathered by an organization (or individual) specifically for a new purpose are known as *primary data*. Primary data pertaining to health needs can be gathered through focus groups, various types of surveys, community meetings, and interviews. The collection of primary data is both expensive and time consuming, but it is invaluable for refining, reaffirming, or revising the information gained through analysis of secondary data. Primary data can be vital for understanding a community's needs, especially if gaps exist in the secondary data collected.

Gathering community input is an IRS-regulated step of the assessment process for not-for-profit hospitals (IRS 2014). The IRS requires that community input from the following three sources be taken into consideration when prioritizing significant health needs:

- At least one representative of a state, regional, or local governmental health department with knowledge of the health needs of the community

- Members of medically underserved, low-income, and minority populations in the community served by the hospital facility, or individuals or organizations serving or representing the interests of such populations
- Written comments from the community regarding the most recently conducted CHNA report and the most recently adopted implementation strategy

Identify Community Input Sources

To begin collecting community input, the Task Force thought about engaging the people who are closely involved in how the community lives, works, learns, worships, and plays. The three hospitals collaborated on the community input plan, and they chose to leverage the partnerships each facility already had in place to collect the input efficiently.

The Task Force developed a list of experts and stakeholders in the community who could be interviewed, keeping in mind that the focus of the assessment is on the health needs of Franklin and Oso County residents. These interviewees were selected because of the valuable insights they could provide into the community's health needs. The Task Force had a long list of potential interviewees, but the time frame required that the list be limited to ten to twelve individuals. The Task Force had to select its subjects carefully to reach multiple perspectives.

In addition, the Task Force also planned focus groups and a community survey, while also looking for other qualitative data that could be integrated into the assessment.

Methods of Gathering Community Input (Primary Data Collection)

Community input can be gathered through a variety of techniques, many of which are described in the University of Kansas's Community Tool Box (available at http://ctb.ku.edu/en). Ultimately, the Oak Grove Task Force decided to focus on the following three:

- *Interviews.* The Task Force chose to interview ten executives of local public and private agencies, including public health departments, schools, two YMCAs, and several community service organizations. These half-hour conversations took place by telephone and were led by researchers from a partner organization who took notes. Participants, many of whom had responded to interview requests for the previous needs assessment cycle, appreciated that the three hospitals were working together on this cycle's CHNA; the collaboration saved them from having to sit through three separate interviews.
- *Focus groups.* The Oak Grove coalition convened ten focus groups, consisting of 8 to 12 members each. Two of the focus groups were for local adolescents in Oso County's largest high school, and two were for Franklin County's largest high school; these focus groups were organized through a partnership with the Department of Education. One focus group of older adults was arranged by the Area Agency on Aging. Another two focused on engaging Hispanic/Latino

community members across the entire service area. Three other focus groups included residents in specific zip codes in the community that had been identified, through secondary data analysis, as having high socioeconomic need. For all the focus groups, questions were prepared ahead of time, but they were individualized and refined for the specifics of each group. The focus groups were led by an experienced facilitator from the partner health department.

- *Community survey.* The Task Force distributed an online survey to the community through the hospital's partners. The purpose of this additional data collection effort was to reach subpopulations for which secondary data were lacking, as well as to further explore areas that stood out as particularly challenging, expensive, or addressable to select subgroups. The survey was developed in Spanish as well as English, so it could reach the Spanish-speaking population (a number of zip codes in the service area had high percentages of people who speak Spanish rather than English at home). Participation in the survey was incentivized with an online raffle for people willing to provide an email address or phone number. The budget for this effort came directly from the Oak Grove Task Force.

These methods are summarized in exhibit 3.5. No single community input tool is better than another. The right tools are those that support the organization, match the skill set, and achieve results within the available budget. Most often, a combination of community input tools is best.

The Oak Grove Task Force created a list of themes for the analysis of the primary data. It engaged researchers from the local university to assist with the data analysis, given that analyzing qualitative data can be complicated and time consuming. Moreover,

EXHIBIT 3.5
Summary Table of Primary Data Collection Methods

Community Input Method	Question Format	Example Questions
Interview	Open-ended	What are the major health needs/issues you see in the community? Who in your community appears to struggle the most with these issues you have identified? How do these issues affect their lives?
Focus group	Specific to the group characteristic or service area	What conditions in your community might prevent someone from accessing healthcare? What role do you think a hospital should have in addressing these needs?
Survey	Demographic and health perceptions and behaviors	Where (i.e., in what zip code) do you currently live? What is your profession? (Check box.) How would you rate your health today?

the Task Force wanted all the data supporting the CHNA to be perceived by the community stakeholders as valid. The list of themes included the following:

- Health needs/issues (subthemes include access to health services, transportation, heart disease, obesity, oral health, nutrition, diabetes, and social environment)
- Barriers to healthcare
- Disparities (subthemes include racial/ethnic disparity, age disparity, gender disparity, and geographic disparity)
- Community resources and assets
- Advice for future planning
- Community priorities

The topics most frequently discussed by the focus groups, interviewees, and survey respondents included mental health and mental disorders, substance abuse, obesity, access to health services, transportation, teen and adolescent health, and poverty.

Step 4: Prioritize Needs

Even though a community may have many significant health needs, an organization often only has the capacity to address a subset of those needs. Thus, the needs must be prioritized based on established criteria. If stakeholders are to be involved in setting priorities, a systematic process must be used to apply the criteria to the range of identified needs. Moreover, the IRS requires not-for-profit hospitals to report how needs identified by the CHNA have been prioritized.

The Oak Grove Task Force considered a list of possible reasons that a health problem might be regarded as a high priority. It also recognized that the two not-for-profit hospitals did not need to address the same problems. The Task Force's list of possible reasons to prioritize a need identified by the CHNA included the following:

- Alignment with the facility's strengths/priorities/mission
- Magnitude—the number of people affected by the problem
- Severity—the rate or risk of morbidity and mortality
- Opportunity to intervene at prevention level
- Opportunity for partnership
- Potential for addressing disparities of subgroups
- Existing resources and programs to address the problem
- Potential solution that could impact multiple problems
- Feasibility of intervention
- Availability of evidence-based approaches to address the problem
- Importance of the problem to the community

- Economic burden on the community
- Consequences of not intervening
- Evaluation of progress made since the last CHNA

As a group, the Task Force chose the following prioritization criteria:

- Opportunity for partnership
- Availability of evidence-based approaches
- Existing resources and programs to address the problem
- Importance of the problem to the community, based on the findings from the primary data collection activities

The Task Force decided to invite stakeholders involved in community health improvement efforts—particularly those working with youth, schools, and underserved neighborhoods—to participate in the upcoming prioritization session. The Task Force then deliberated upon which method they would use for the prioritization process. The methods considered are described in exhibit 3.6. To be as objective as possible, the Task Force decided to use a prioritization matrix; they wanted to ensure that each focus area was reviewed systematically according to the prioritization criteria selected.

EXHIBIT 3.6
Methods of
Prioritization

Method	Description
Dot method / dotmocracy	A quick and simple method that works well with large groups. Individuals are given a set number of dots (stickers) and vote for the needs that they believe meet the established criteria.
Multivoting technique	A great method to narrow a lot of options down to a few, by allowing individuals to vote for a set number of topics in each round. After each round is completed, only the top results are included in the next round.
Nominal group technique	An ideal method for small groups of decision makers who have a deep knowledge of the selection criteria. This method involves generating topics, recording topics, discussing topics, and then voting on topics.
Strategy grid	A good method for using only two criteria with groups of decision makers who have a deep knowledge of the criteria and the issues. The strategy grid allows decision makers to focus on topics that will have the best results.
Prioritization matrix	A good method for small to medium-sized groups using multiple criteria to select priorities. Participants systematically analyze each priority based on the criteria.
Paired comparison	An advanced method whereby participants compare pairs of health needs based on different criteria using a matrix.
Hanlon method	A complex method that incorporates baseline data into an objective analysis of the criteria and the different health needs.

After reviewing findings from both the primary and secondary data, the Task Force arrived at the following list of top health needs to further prioritize:

- Exercise, nutrition, and weight
- Access to health services
- Transportation
- Heart disease and stroke
- Substance abuse
- Cancer
- Mental health and mental disorders
- Teen and adolescent health
- Poverty

After conducting the prioritization session, the Task Force determined that the top three priorities to address would be the following:

- Exercise, nutrition, and weight
- Access to health services, including transportation issues
- Substance abuse

Step 5: Inventory Existing Programs and Resources

Now that the significant health needs had been prioritized, the Task Force set out to map community assets—which is shorthand for identifying existing programs and community resources relevant to each priority need. If one or more organizations in the community are already engaged in addressing a given need, a hospital or other partner agency might determine either that its involvement is not needed or that it should join the existing efforts; it would not duplicate or repeat programs. In reporting to the IRS, a hospital might justify not acting on a need of high priority by explaining that other organizations in the community were already focusing on that need. (Note: Asset mapping is the subject of case study 2.)

Step 6: Develop an Implementation Strategy

This next phase involves the following:

- Exploring the evidence base (e.g., the Community Guide, What Works for Health) to learn about programs that have been shown to be effective in addressing a given problem with a given subgroup of the population
- Engaging institutional leadership, as well as partners and other stakeholders, if desired, in selecting the most appropriate strategies to implement
- Developing a concrete framework for implementation and evaluation—which the IRS refers to as the implementation strategy

Final Report

The Oak Grove CHNA Task Force completed steps 1 through 5 over a six-month period. The description of the process and the findings could then be compiled into the CHNA report. The report's table of contents is shown in exhibit 3.7. A set of tips for preparing a final CHNA is provided in exhibit 3.8.

EXHIBIT 3.7
Table of Contents for the Oak Grove Community Health Needs Assessment

Oak Grove Community Hospital
2016 Community Health Needs Assessment

Table of Contents

1. **Executive Summary**
   a. Introduction
   b. Summary of Findings
   c. Prioritized Areas

2. **Introduction**
   a. Oak Grove Community Hospital
      i. Service Area
      ii. Team
   b. Collaboration

3. **Evaluation of Progress Since Prior CHNA**
   a. Priority Health Topics from Previous CHNA
   b. Community Feedback from Previous CHNA and Implementation Plan

4. **Methodology**
   a. Overview
   b. Secondary Data Sources and Analysis
   c. Primary Data Collection and Analysis
   d. Data Considerations
   e. Prioritization

5. **Demographics**

6. **Data Synthesis**

7. **Prioritized Significant Health Needs**

8. **Nonprioritized Significant Health Needs**

9. **Other Findings**

10. **Conclusion**

11. **Appendices**
    a. Oak Grove Impact Report
    b. Secondary Data Methodology
    c. Primary Data Methodology
    d. Prioritization Tools
    e. Community Resources

EXHIBIT 3.8
Tips for a Final
CHNA Report

- Include secondary data from local, state, and national sources that are validated, reliable, and available at granular geographies.
- Indicate when, where, and how the community input was obtained and analyzed.
- Include the names of the organizations that provided input into the CHNA, and summarize the nature and extent of that input.
- Make sure to describe the medically underserved, low-income, or minority populations being represented by the individual or organization providing input.
- In the event that a hospital solicits but cannot obtain community input from a certain source, the CHNA report must describe the hospital's efforts to solicit that input.
- Make sure to document the prioritization process and criteria used, and include the results.

The Task Force reviewed IRS guidelines to ensure that all components had been included and documented according to IRS requirements. All three hospitals could use the same CHNA report, although only the two nonprofit hospitals had to submit it to the IRS. The implementation strategy—which explains what each hospital intended to do with the information to create or revise programs to address the identified health needs—would be done independently by each hospital. Despite having a common CHNA, the actions taken by each hospital in response to identified needs might be different.

The two nonprofit hospitals will need to take additional steps. The completed CHNA must be submitted to each hospital's board for approval. Once approved, it must be shared for public comment, both by posting it on each hospital's website and by having paper copies available upon request.

The public availability of the document, as well as the extensive efforts the Task Force made to involve representatives of the community, meant that other health and related organizations in Oak Grove could use the CHNA information for their own program purposes. Beyond just meeting IRS regulations, the combined CHNA would serve the community and hopefully instill good will and collaboration among the many stakeholders who had been represented in its process.

Questions

Fact and Data Analysis Questions

1. What is the purpose/spirit/intention of the IRS guidelines requiring not-for-profit hospitals to conduct a community health needs assessment every three years?
2. Why do both primary and secondary data need to be collected? How do primary and secondary data complement each other?
3. How does a not-for-profit hospital define its service area for IRS reporting purposes?

4. What factors or attributes are important to consider when gathering secondary data?
5. Name two examples of ways in which secondary data can be analyzed.
6. What is the function of community input in a CHNA?
7. Why should more than one type of community input method be used?
8. Give one strength and one weakness for each of the following methods of community input: focus groups, interviews, surveys, and public forums.
9. Why must hospitals prioritize health needs?
10. What are some methods for identifying priorities in an open process?

Discussion Questions

1. What are the advantages and disadvantages of two or more community organizations working together on a CHNA?
2. How can social determinants of health inform a hospital's plan to address significant health needs?
3. Aside from IRS requirements, why does a hospital or other healthcare organization need to consider disparities among the subpopulations it serves?
4. As a national policy, is "community benefit" effective in improving the health of communities? Why or why not?

References

Conduent Healthy Communities Institute. 2018. "What Is the SocioNeeds Index Ranking and How Is It Determined?" Published December 11. https://help.healthycities.org/hc/en-us/articles/220328707-What-is-the-SocioNeeds-Index-ranking-and-how-is-it-determined.

Health Services Research Information Central. 2019. "Community Benefit / Community Health Needs Assessment." Updated June 3. www.nlm.nih.gov/hsrinfo/community_benefit.html.

Internal Revenue Service (IRS). 2014. "Additional Requirements for Charitable Hospitals; Community Health Needs Assessments for Charitable Hospitals; Requirement of a Section 4959 Excise Tax Return and Time for Filing the Return." Published December 31. www.federalregister.gov/documents/2014/12/31/2014-30525/additional-requirements-for-charitable-hospitals-community-health-needs-assessments-for-charitable.

Useful Resources

- Association for Community Health Improvement—Community Health Assessment Toolkit (www.healthycommunities.org/Resources/toolkit.shtml#.W0j5RsgnY_U)

- Catholic Health Association of the United States—Community Benefit Overview (www.chausa.org/communitybenefit/community-benefit)
- Centers for Disease Control and Prevention—Community Guide (www.thecommunityguide.org)
- Centers for Disease Control and Prevention—Community Health Improvement Navigator (www.cdc.gov/chinav/)
- Centers for Disease Control and Prevention—Prioritization (www.cdc.gov/nphpsp/documents/Prioritization%20section%20from%20APEXPH%20in%20Practice.pdf)
- Healthy People (www.healthypeople.gov)
- Internal Revenue Service Requirements for Charitable Hospitals (www.federalregister.gov/documents/2014/12/31/2014-30525/additional-requirements-for-charitable-hospitals-community-health-needs-assessments-for-charitable)
- MindTools—Prioritization (www.mindtools.com/pages/article/newHTE_92.htm)
- National Institutes of Health—Community Benefit / Community Health Needs Assessment (www.nlm.nih.gov/hsrinfo/community_benefit.html)
- University of Kansas Community Tool Box (https://ctb.ku.edu/en)

SOCIAL DETERMINANTS OF HEALTH

The World Health Organization (WHO) defines the *social determinants of health* (SDoH) as "the conditions in which people are born, grow, work, live, and age, and the wider set of forces and systems shaping the conditions of daily life. These forces and systems include economic policies and systems, development agendas, social norms, social policies and political systems" (WHO 2019b). The SDoH include demographic and economic conditions, such as income, education, and race; environmental factors, such as housing, walkability, and transportation; and public policies, such as clean water enforcement, recycling, and priorities for bond issues.

Healthy People (2019a), a program of the United States Department of Health and Human Services, explains SDoH similarly:

> Social determinants of health are conditions in the environments in which people live, learn, work, play, worship, and age that affect a wide range of health, functioning, and quality-of-life outcomes and risks. Conditions (e.g., social, economic, and physical) in these various environments and settings (e.g., school, church, workplace, and neighborhood) have been referred to as "place." In addition to the more material attributes of "place," the patterns of social engagement and sense of security and well-being are also affected by where people live.

The WHO convened a Commission on Social Determinants of Health from 2005 to 2008. Chaired by Sir Michael Marmott, the commission gathered evidence about the impact social factors have on health and health inequities. The commission's final report generated worldwide visibility of the importance of SDoH on the health of individuals, select subpopulations, and entire communities (WHO 2008). The WHO's Sustainable Development Goals (SDGs) provide a comprehensive blueprint for human development and for systematically addressing the SDoH throughout the world (WHO 2019a).

SDoH stand in contrast to individual risk factors, which might be the result of genetics, and which tend to be less subject to intentional modification. SDoH can be manifest in cultural norms, conditions of the natural environment, or government policies, and they can have a powerful impact on health-promoting behaviors, health statuses, and the potential success of interventions. One of the overarching goals of Healthy People 2020 is to "create social and physical environments that promote good health for all" (Healthy People 2019b), which emphasizes the breadth and significance of SDoH.

The two cases in this section address SDoH from different perspectives. Case 4 focuses on a health system's realization that treating individual patients who are in emergency situations does not bring about long-term solutions for the individuals or for the community. Rather, community-wide actions are needed to address the problems that cause homelessness, which in turn contribute to poor health status, human suffering, and inappropriate or unnecessary utilization of scarce healthcare resources.

Case 5 describes a health problem discovered by the healthcare system but caused by adverse housing conditions, combined with a lack of health literacy by clients and cultural competence by providers. Public health experts, healthcare providers, immigration officers, and a variety of advocacy groups came together to solve the immediate problem and to propose long-term solutions at the public policy level.

References

Healthy People. 2019a. "Social Determinants of Health." Accessed January 31. www.healthypeople.gov/2020/topics-objectives/topic/social-determinants-of-health.

———. 2019b. "The Vision, Mission, and Goals of Healthy People 2020." Accessed June 4. www.healthypeople.gov/sites/default/files/HP2020Framework.pdf.

World Health Organization (WHO). 2019a. "Health in the SDG Era." Accessed June 4. www.who.int/topics/sustainable-development-goals/test/sdg-banner.jpg.

———. 2019b. "Social Determinants of Health." Accessed January 31. www.who.int/social_determinants/en/.

———. 2008. *Closing the Gap in a Generation: Health Equity Through Action on the Social Determinants of Health*. Geneva, Switzerland: World Health Organization.

SOCIAL DETERMINANTS OF HEALTH: SHELTERING PEOPLE EXPERIENCING HOMELESSNESS IN VERMONT

Penrose Jackson, Margaret Rost, Margaret Bozik, and Chris Donnelly

Note: This case is based on a real experience. The description of the history and the early statistics are accurate. The management challenge and other details have been created for pedagogical purposes; they are realistic but fictitious.

Acknowledgments: The authors would like to acknowledge and thank the following individuals for their contributions to institutional efforts to help those experiencing homelessness and to the preparation of this case study: Tammy Boudah, Dr. Steven Grant, Dr. Stephen Leffler, Dean Pallozzi, and Rick Vincent.

Case at a Glance

Overarching theme	The focus of this chapter is to apply a not-for-profit hospital's community benefit activities to address the effect of social determinants of health, specifically the experience of homelessness, on health service utilization.
Learning objectives	• Apply the social determinants of health and Ecological Model of Health concepts to community health programs. • Analyze the health status of a defined population and trends over time. • Explain the causes and characteristics of homelessness. • Evaluate the business case for a health organization being involved with its community. • Differentiate activities done by nonprofit hospitals for "community benefit" from those done for other reasons. • Critique the elements that make interorganizational collaboration effective over time. • Relate community analytics to institutional performance.

Key terms	• Backbone institution • Community benefit • Ecological Model of Health • Homelessness • Housing and Urban Development (HUD) vouchers • Internal Revenue Service Form 990, Schedule H • Nonprofit/not-for-profit organization • Population health • Section 8 housing • Social determinants of health (SDoH) • Tax exemption • Upstream factors
Management competencies	Managing community benefit, social determinants of health, governance of coalitions
Population/subgroup	People experiencing homelessness
Health issue or condition	Multiple chronic conditions, mental and behavioral health challenges

Management Challenge

Improving the health of the community has always been an integral part of the vision of the University of Vermont Medical Center (UVM MC 2019a)—"Working together, we improve people's lives." With that in mind, UVM MC launched an initiative to respond to the needs of the people in its community who are experiencing homelessness. Initially, the leadership approved the funding; several years later, however, the senior leadership has changed. The new leaders need to be educated about the Ecological Model of Health (see exhibit 4.1), as well as about how social determinants of health (SDoH) affect the medical center. The new leaders need to understand the rationale for UVM MC being in the "housing" business.

EXHIBIT 4.1
The Ecological
Model—A
Framework for
Prevention

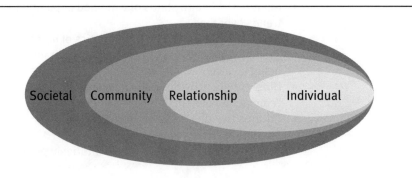

Source: Centers for Disease Control and Prevention (2019).

UVM MC's vice president for community engagement is trying to create a presentation about the impact of SDoH that will explain the relevance of the housing initiatives to the organization's mission, financial status, community benefit requirement, and clinical operations.

Background

Vermont (see exhibit 4.2) is one of the smallest states in the United States. In 2018, it had an estimated population of 626,000 (US Census Bureau 2019). Vermont's capital, Montpelier, is the least-populated state capital in the country. UVM MC is in Burlington, Vermont's most populated city, about 45 miles south of the US–Canadian border

EXHIBIT 4.2
Map of Vermont

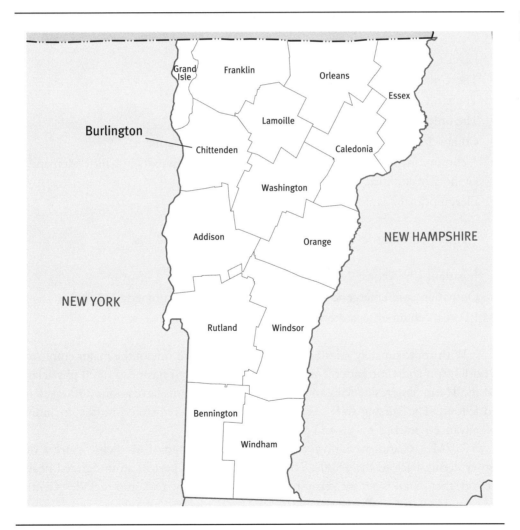

Source: Adapted from US Geological Survey.

and 95 miles from Montreal, the second largest city in Canada. The terrain of Vermont is primarily mountainous with dense forests. The temperature ranges from –7 degrees Fahrenheit in the winter months to 79 degrees in the summer. The demographic and economic characteristics of the population can be gleaned from US Census data or County Health Rankings. Vermont's homeless population is disproportionately large compared to that of other states.

University of Vermont Medical Center

UVM MC, a nonprofit 501(c)(3) organization, is one of 138 academic medical centers in the United States (UVM MC 2019b). It is a regional referral center for approximately 1 million people in Vermont and northern New York. UVM MC has more than 30 patient care sites and more than 100 outreach clinics and programs, with tertiary services covering every major area of medicine. Its services include the following:

- Level 1 Trauma Center
- The University of Vermont Children's Hospital
- The University of Vermont Cancer Center
- The only neonatal intensive care unit in Vermont
- Comprehensive cardiovascular services and stroke treatment
- A community hospital for approximately 160,000 residents in Chittenden and Grand Isle counties, Vermont
- Eleven primary care clinics in Vermont

Its patient statistics for the most recent year are as follows:

- Inpatient admissions: 22,100
- Outpatient and emergency department (ED) visits combined: 375,000
- ED visits counted separately: 59,500

With approximately 7,500 employees, UVM MC is one of the major employers in Burlington and Chittenden counties. The medical staff has nearly 800 physicians, and the 16 training residencies and 23 fellowship programs have about 300 residents and fellows. The nursing staff has approximately 1,750 registered nurses, including 160 advanced practice nurses and physician assistants.

UVM MC and the University of Vermont College of Medicine share a rich history dating back to the 1800s. The medical center is part of an integrated health network that extends across Vermont and northern New York and includes Central Vermont Medical Center (Berlin, VT), UVM Champlain Valley Physicians Hospital (Plattsburgh, NY), Elizabethtown Community Hospital (Elizabethtown, NY), and Alice Hyde Medical Center (Malone, NY).

Housing Challenges in UVM MC's Health Service Area

UVM MC and other community organizations have recognized affordable, stable housing as a crucial need for the individuals they serve. Every community health needs assessment (CHNA) since the 1980s has listed "affordable housing" as a top need. From a clinical perspective, providers at UVM MC have recognized that their patients experience healthcare challenges related to inadequate housing (Institute of Medicine Committee on Health Care for Homeless People 1988).

If patients are discharged from the hospital without a safe and reliable place to store medication or simply to sleep, trips back to the emergency room are difficult to avoid. Lack of housing has been shown to lead to the following:

- Increased rates of physical trauma, chronic diseases, dental issues, behavioral health problems, and exposure
- Reduced access to primary care and reduced ability to self-manage health and wellbeing
- Inappropriate use of services—80 percent of ED visits by patients experiencing homelessness could be prevented through primary care treatments

In 2012, the Champlain Housing Trust (CHT), a community land trust and affordable housing provider, surveyed community partners while developing its three-year strategic plan. One recurring theme that CHT heard from partners was that it was not doing enough to address the growing homelessness challenge in Chittenden County, the state's most populous county. Affordable housing continued to rank as a prevalent need in UVM MC's 2013 and 2016 CHNAs.

According to the annual *Point-In-Time* count of homelessness in Vermont, the problem has worsened in the past decade; chronic homelessness more than doubled between 2010 and 2012 (Vermont Coalition to End Homelessness and Chittenden County Homeless Alliance 2019). Chittenden County in particular suffers from a dearth of affordable housing (see exhibit 4.3). The rental vacancy rate has ranged from less than 1 percent to 2.5 percent in recent years, with resultant high rents in comparison to wages.

EXHIBIT 4.3
Vermont Housing Data

	Chittenden County	Grand Isle County	Vermont
Median monthly housing cost	$1,139	$989	$913
Rental vacancy rate	2.2%	8.2%	4.2%
Total housing units	67,523	5,117	326,812
Percent of units where gross rent is more than 35% of household income	43.6%	40.3%	41%

Source: Data from the US Census Bureau (www.census.gov).

Call to Action

In 2012, three people who had been experiencing homelessness died from exposure, and the tragedy spurred state leadership to act. Vermont Governor Peter Shumlin directed the Agency of Human Services (AHS) to create a flexible program that would prevent people from freezing to death (Moats 2012). The AHS created a motel voucher program that grew to over $4 million per year, but the agency had few tools to ensure that the motels were safe or that people housed in them were better off.

Seeking a better solution to the problem, CHT convinced the state and several local social service providers to try a new approach. In November 2013, CHT purchased a 59-room motel in a suburb of Burlington, rebranded it Harbor Place, and secured promises from community agencies, including UVM MC, to send clients there when needed (Hughes 2018). The offer of rooms at a 60 percent discount (relative to the median cost of a commercial motel room) promised immediate savings to the state. Harbor Place also provided on-site case management to help residents to get back on their feet more quickly. The cost structure of Harbor Place made it an acceptable business operation for CHT, so long-term continuity was incorporated into the business plan.

UVM MC had long used local motels for patients who no longer needed inpatient care but who lacked a safe home, or any home, to return to. Harbor Place marked the beginning of a collaboration between UVM MC and CHT that would only grow stronger over time and have more impact than either organization could have imagined. A variety of institutions in the greater Burlington community took part in the effort to address the problem of homelessness, as shown in exhibit 4.4.

Harbor Place has 39 single units and 20 one- and two-room units with kitchenettes. UVM MC discharges patients to Harbor Place if they have no safe housing alternative. In the first three years of operation, 168 patients were discharged there, and the average length of stay was 13.1 days.

As shown in exhibit 4.5, Harbor Place has been effective in reducing the number of patient encounters and the direct costs for people experiencing homelessness. Tammy Boudah, a member of the Howard Center's Street Outreach Team, has witnessed improvements among the population she works with since Harbor Place's inception. Tammy states:

> Healthcare has become more accessible as individuals experiencing homelessness can access preventive and acute medical services. For example, adults in their 50s living on the street or in shelters are unable to prepare for procedures such as colonoscopies, thus will not get them, leading to more serious conditions down the road. Additionally, Harbor Place gives people experiencing homelessness a chance to recover from illnesses. For example, before Harbor

Place, individuals discharged from the hospital with pneumonia would either return to the street or bounce back and forth between a shelter and a day station, having little opportunity to rest and fully recuperate.

Harbor Place's success deepened the partnerships among the participating community organizations. Several partners moved forward with a second initiative, Beacon Apartments, to permanently house residents who had been chronically homeless and medically vulnerable. Like Harbor Place, Beacon Apartments is a renovated motel. The facility has 19 permanent housing units, with on-site social services provided by the Community Health Centers of Burlington and their homeless healthcare program, Safe Harbor Clinic. UVM MC has helped fund these services.

EXHIBIT 4.4
Key Institutions in the Greater Burlington Community

Partner	Role
Champlain Housing Trust (CHT)	Conceptualized Harbor Place by bringing together partners, securing financing and long-term leases, and purchasing and renovating the property; also serves as a liaison with the state.
The UVM Medical Center	Provided funding to CHT for operating reserve; purchases bed nights for approximately 45 patients per year.
Vermont Agency of Human Services / Department for Children and Families	Funded operating reserves, giving access to 30 of the rooms at Harbor Place.
Fanny Allen Foundation	Provided a $25,000 grant toward operating reserve for Harbor Place.
United Way of Northwest Vermont	Provided $50,000 toward operating reserve.
Vermont Housing and Conservation Board	Provided $265,000 for acquisition and rehabilitation of the property.
Vermont Community Loan Fund	Provided a $1.7 million loan to finance the purchase of the motel.
Howard Center (designated mental health agency)	Provides on-site mental health and substance-abuse counseling services; refers clients to Harbor Place.
Safe Harbor Health Care / Community Health Center of Burlington (Federally Qualified Health Center)	Provides on-site case management and medical services.
Champlain Valley Office of Economic Opportunity	Oversees case management at Harbor Place, as well as providing direct support staffing.

EXHIBIT 4.5
Harbor Place
Patient
Intervention
Study

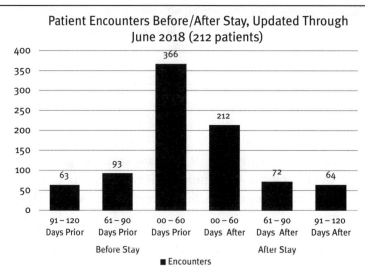

Patient Encounters Before/After Stay, Updated Through June 2018 (212 patients)

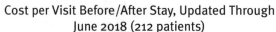

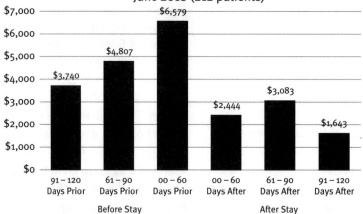

Cost per Visit Before/After Stay, Updated Through June 2018 (212 patients)

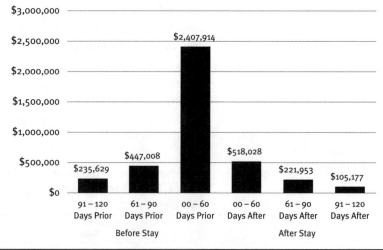

Direct Costs Before/After Stay, Updated Through June 2018 (212 patients)

Source: Used with permission from University of Vermont Medical Center.

EXHIBIT 4.6
Beacon
Apartments
Patient
Intervention
Study

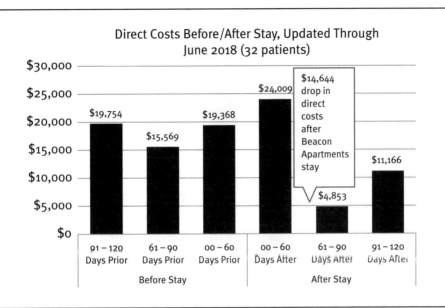

Direct Costs Before/After Stay, Updated Through June 2018 (32 patients)

Source: Used with permission from University of Vermont Medical Center.

As illustrated in exhibit 4.6, the number of patient encounters and direct costs for patients have decreased since patients moved to Beacon Apartments.

The positive impact of Beacon Apartments is reflected not only in the collected data but also in the stories shared by residents. One man, who was homeless in the aftermath of a divorce, moved into Beacon Apartments after working proactively with a case manager from Community Health Centers of Burlington's Safe Harbor Clinic. Since then, he says things have changed dramatically:

> Just knowing that, when I get through my door, I can close it, shut the world out, and have all the comforts of home. . . . It's just nice to sit back and not worry about where I'm going to bounce to next.

Collaborations have continued, in part because of the shared vision and ongoing communication among the partner agencies. CHT acquired a third motel property, Bel Aire, to further combat chronic homelessness. UVM MC provided the capital for CHT to purchase and renovate the motel into eight apartments, and it pledged to pay the Community Health Centers of Burlington for medical and social work supports. Five of the eight apartments are available as permanent housing for people who have been chronically homeless. The remaining three apartments, with seven bedrooms total, are master leased to UVM MC to provide medical respite to people who are discharged from the hospital and have nowhere else to go. Both the data and the stories from people involved indicate that Bel Aire has served as a helpful bridge to recovery for patients while they explore longer-term housing solutions (see exhibit 4.7).

Findings from the 2019 *Point-in-Time* report (see exhibit 4.8) show improvements in homelessness statistics in the years since these collaborations have been initiated.

EXHIBIT 4.7
Bel Aire Patient
Intervention
Study

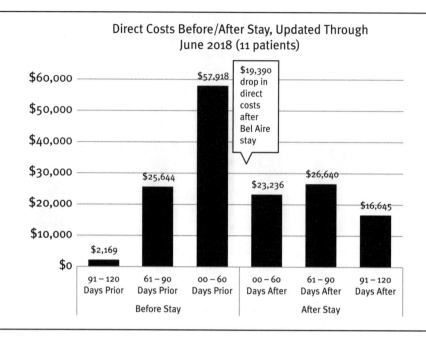

Direct Costs Before/After Stay, Updated Through June 2018 (11 patients)

- $2,169 — 91–120 Days Prior
- $25,644 — 61–90 Days Prior
- $57,918 — 00–60 Days Prior
- $23,236 — 00–60 Days After
- $26,640 — 61–90 Days After
- $16,645 — 91–120 Days After

$19,390 drop in direct costs after Bel Aire stay

Before Stay / After Stay

Source: Used with permission from University of Vermont Medical Center.

EXHIBIT 4.8
Vermont
Homelessness
Statistics

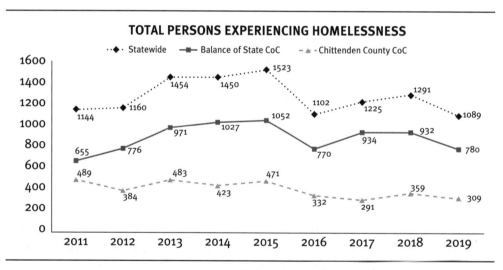

TOTAL PERSONS EXPERIENCING HOMELESSNESS

···◆··· Statewide   ■ Balance of State CoC   ▲ Chittenden County CoC

	2011	2012	2013	2014	2015	2016	2017	2018	2019
Statewide	1144	1160	1454	1450	1523	1102	1225	1291	1089
Balance of State CoC	655	776	971	1027	1052	770	934	932	780
Chittenden County CoC	489	384	483	423	471	332	291	359	309

Note: CoC = Continuum of Care.
Source: Data from Vermont Coalition to End Homelessness and Chittenden County Homeless Alliance (2019).

Coordinated Entry

An integral part of these collaborations' success has been the implementation of Coordinated Entry, a system for streamlining access to housing supports and resources in Chittenden County. The system was developed to evaluate people experiencing homelessness and match them with appropriate services, using a standardized, scored assessment based on vulnerability, sustainability, and length of homelessness.

Candidates for Harbor Place, Beacon Apartments, and Bel Aire, as well as other services, are identified in acute care settings, through social service agencies, and in the community at large, and frontline workers in these settings administer the assessments. Candidates who are deemed eligible are placed on the community master list and referred to the appropriate committee for housing placement. Individuals are placed based on their scores:

1. With a high score, a person is referred to the Permanent Supportive Housing committee for ongoing specialized rental subsidy (Shelter Plus Care or Mental Health) and support services.
2. With a medium score, the person is referred to the Community Housing Resource committee for ongoing mainstream rental subsidy (Section 8), plus time-limited and episodic support services.
3. With a low score, the person is referred to the Housing Resource Team for short-term rental subsidy and short-term support services.

Once in a committee, the person is assigned a housing navigator to help with filling out paperwork and finding an apartment.

Challenges

Many moving parts have been involved in the execution of these housing programs. UVM MC and its partners faced several challenges throughout the process, including the following:

- The town in which Harbor Place is located initially objected to the zoning classification for short-term housing and attempted to shut down the operation. Representatives from CHT, UVM MC, and other community organizations came together to articulate the importance of the facility and were successful in obtaining approval for the project's implementation.
- Finding the right individuals to staff the housing facilities can be challenging. Services at Bel Aire were delayed as the partner organizations needed more time to hire the on-site case manager.
- The interest and commitment of partner agencies over time can be affected by leadership turnover in the various agencies, the advocacy efforts of those who champion the homeless, and the evolution of UVM MC's own strategic directions. Educating the board of UVM MC, as well as the other organizations in town, is an essential element for sustainability.
- The IRS has continued to change the reporting requirements for community benefit. Schedule H of Form 990 has grown from four pages in 2008 to as many as 75 pages for some of UVM MC's peer organizations.

Impact on UVM MC

One of the initial reasons UVM MC partnered on housing initiatives was to further its move toward management of the health of the community it serves, part of the long-term goal of succeeding in a value-based financing structure for healthcare. An equally important reason was fulfilling its contribution to the community and meeting the IRS requirements for not-for-profit hospitals (to be reported on Form 990, Schedule H).

The board of UVM MC, like the board of any nonprofit healthcare entity, is constantly challenged to balance mission with financial stability. UVM MC seeks to be transparent with its partners, its patients, and its community. Just meeting regulatory requirements is not sufficient; UVM MC knows that its stakeholders will see its community benefit activities, and it wants their reaction to be positive.

Conclusions and Lessons Learned

Fortunately, doing the right thing for its community has also proven to be a smart investment for UVM MC, as the healthcare system transitions from a fee-for-service approach to a structure that rewards efforts to keep people healthy. People who have affordable, quality housing have improved access to medical care and better health outcomes overall. UVM MC helps patients find housing so they can focus on healing.

Since 2013, UVM MC has partnered with Vermont's state government and private nonprofits on a variety of projects and initiatives to address local housing needs. These collaborations have contributed to a nearly 50 percent reduction in homelessness in Chittenden County between 2013 and 2018, coupled with savings of $1 million in healthcare expenses over the same period.

Lessons learned about effective collaboration among multiple organizations serving the same community include the following:

1. Proactively identify the community-wide gap to solve.
2. Garner support from finance leaders by focusing on initiatives with trackable measures that link cost savings.
3. Create a bilateral outreach strategy to implementation and influencer partners, especially when targeting stigmatized populations.
4. Hardwire clear communications channels, such as quarterly leadership meetings, to systematically break down silos.
5. Invest in building strong ties with community health centers and other frontline entities, which are best positioned to face the realities of vulnerable populations.

Now, UVM MC's vice president of community engagement is trying to decide what approach she should take to educate the new executives about care for the homeless, the rationale for the medical center to become involved with social determinants of health, and the financial implications of the housing initiatives. What data can she share? What rationale can she offer to persuade the senior leaders to invest in additional SDoH programs in the future? What should be UVM MC's priorities for providing community benefit?

Questions

Fact and Data Analysis Questions

1. What are the demographic and economic characteristics of the counties served by UVM MC?
2. Who defines the word *homeless*? Do definitions vary across states, cities, or other boundaries?
3. What is the relationship between homelessness and health status?
4. What are social determinants of health? What is the Ecological Model of Health? How do the two relate?
5. How might UVM MC analyze its patients to identify homelessness as a problem? What other population groups might have health challenges stemming from social determinants of health? How might these issues be identified from patient records?
6. In reporting to the IRS on Form 990, Schedule H, how would UVM MC define its "community"?
7. What part of the program to address homelessness is reported on the UVM MC Form 990, Schedule H, as community benefit? How are social determinants of health recognized on Schedule H?
8. What percentage of the homeless population will be accommodated by the housing developed by UVM MC and its partners?

Discussion Questions

1. Buying or building housing for homeless patients will not in itself solve a healthcare system's challenges in taking care of homeless patients. What else is needed?
2. Construction or purchase of a physical plant is an expensive endeavor. What else could the health system have done with its resources to address the problem of homelessness in its community? Why was the physical plant the option of choice?
3. What public organizations have a responsibility to provide for the homeless? What private agencies are likely to be involved in addressing issues related to

homelessness in a community? What is the role of the health system as a leader of community initiatives?

4. Does having a large homeless population affect the health status of the rest of the community?

5. Draw the organizational chart showing the lines of authority, responsibility, and accountability for the various organizations involved in the first housing initiative. How would you expect these relationships to evolve over time? What management techniques would be useful in coordinating the interaction of the entities?

6. From a financial perspective, how does an organization such as UVM MC decide whether it will pursue a program to benefit the health status of the community or to benefit the financial status of the institution?

7. How might the financial parameters change if the insurance status of those experiencing homelessness changes—for example, if the state Medicaid program changes from fee-for-service to capitation?

8. Critique the use of a screening tool, such as that developed by the Coordinated Entry program, for its strengths and weaknesses in identifying a high-risk population.

References

Centers for Disease Control and Prevention (CDC). 2019. "The Social-Ecological Model: A Framework for Violence Prevention." Accessed June 4. www.cdc.gov/ViolencePrevention/pdf/SEM_Framewrk-a.pdf.

Hughes, M. 2018. "Harbor Place Team Connects Guests, Services and Homes." *Shelburne News*. Published December 1. www.shelburnenews.com/2018/12/01/harbor-place-team-connects-guests-services-homes/.

Institute of Medicine Committee on Health Care for Homeless People. 1988. "Health Problems of Homeless People." Accessed June 5, 2019. www.ncbi.nlm.nih.gov/books/NBK218236/.

Moats, T. 2012. "Shumlin: We Need to House Homeless People." *Barre Montpelier Times Argus*. Published January 26. www.timesargus.com/articles/shumlin-we-need-to-house-homeless-people/.

University of Vermont Medical Center (UVM MC). 2019a. "Mission, Vision & Values." Accessed June 4. www.uvmhealth.org/medcenter/Pages/About-UVM-Medical-Center/Mission-Vision-and-Values.aspx. www.cdc.gov/ViolencePrevention/pdf/SEM_Framewrk-a.pdf.

———. 2019b. "Overview." Accessed June 5. www.uvmhealth.org/medcenter/pages/about-uvm-medical-center/overview.aspx.

US Census Bureau. 2019. "QuickFacts: Vermont." Accessed June 4. https://www.census.gov/quickfacts/VT.

Vermont Coalition to End Homelessness and Chittenden County Homeless Alliance. 2019. *2019 Point-in-Time Count: Everyone Counts, No Matter Where They Live*. Published May. http://helpingtohousevt.org/wp-content/uploads/2019/05/2019-PIT-Report-FINAL.docx.pdf.

Useful Resources

- County Health Rankings (www.countyhealthrankings.org)
- US Department of Housing and Urban Development (www.hud.gov; look for programs available for low-income people)
- US Department of Housing and Urban Development—Continuum of Care Dashboard Reports (www.hudexchange.info/programs/coc/coc-dashboard-reports/?filter_Year=&filter_State=VT&filter_CoC=VT-501&program=CoC&group=Dash)
- VTDigger—Halfway Hotels (https://vtdigger.org/investigations/halfway-hotels/)

LEAD FREE OR DIE: PREVENTING NEW HAMPSHIRE'S WICKED PROBLEM

Rosemary M. Caron

Note: This case is based on actual events that have been adapted for the purposes of class discussion. See Caron et al. (2001) for the original article describing the events.

Acknowledgments: I would like to acknowledge and thank the expert faculty at the Harvard T. H. Chan School of Public Health and my colleagues J. Davis, K. Brown, and A. Batuda for their insightful discussion about the introduction to the case study.

Case at a Glance

Overarching theme	This case focuses on analyzing the impact of social determinants of health on individual health status and evaluating the relevancy of cultural competence to healthcare and prevention; analyzing the evolution of public policy is a secondary focus.
Learning objectives	• Analyze the characteristics of a community. • Define *cultural competence* and describe its effects on the health of a community and defined subpopulations. • Find and apply data to analyze the health status of a community or defined population. • Identify the components of a community's healthcare system. • Apply the social determinants of health and Ecological Model of Health concepts to community health programs. • Analyze the evolution of public policies pertaining to public health prevention initiatives.

Key terms	• Community • Community health • Cultural competence • Epidemiology • Health literacy • Managerial epidemiology • Population • Population health • Public health • Target market
Management competencies	Managerial epidemiology, cultural competence, health literacy, policy analysis
Populations/ subgroups	Children, immigrants
Health issue or condition	Lead poisoning

Management Challenge

A New Hampshire community had an abrupt awakening that lead poisoning was causing serious injury to the area's children and families, and healthcare leaders—including the public health department, physicians, and the academic medical center—realized that something needed to be done immediately. The leaders came together to discuss how the problem could be stopped and what actions should be taken by which organizations. First, they needed a comprehensive analysis of the relevant data.

Background

In late spring, a public health specialist with the City of Manchester (New Hampshire) Health Department (MHD) was investigating the lead-poisoning death of a Sudanese refugee child. Given all the community prevention efforts that have been put in place to address the issue of lead-based paint in older New England homes, how can a child still die of lead poisoning? This question weighed heavily on the minds of the public health professionals.

The child's family consisted of a single Sudanese refugee mother and three siblings. They had been resettled in Manchester because of the death of the husband and the challenges of civil war in their home country. Cultural practices and the mother's illiteracy presented challenges in the gathering of information, but a medical assessment estimated the age range of the children to be from 2 to 12 years.

In early spring, the 2-year-old child had presented to the local emergency department. The mother—communicating through a formerly resettled refugee who spoke an Arabic dialect close to (but not exactly the same as) her own—described flulike symptoms. The child was treated and discharged with a diagnosis of strep throat and vomiting (Caron et al. 2001).

Over the next two weeks, the child's condition deteriorated. The mother returned with the child to the same emergency department, but, following an examination, the medical personnel were unable to determine a diagnosis. The child was then transferred to the state's only tertiary care facility, but she soon became unresponsive. A heavy metal toxicology screen showed a blood lead level 78 times higher than the Centers for Disease Control and Prevention's (CDC's) action level of 5 micrograms per deciliter (Caron et al. 2001; CDC 2019).

Following aggressive treatment using chelation therapy, the child's blood lead level decreased to 14 times the CDC action level. However, the child never regained consciousness. She expired two months after the family had settled into their new home in Manchester (Caron et al. 2001).

Despite a federal ban on lead paint in 1978, lead-based paint remains a significant community health issue for populations in New England. The challenge now is to determine how this child encountered this risk, what implications the case has for the community, and how similar cases can be prevented in the future.

The Environmental Protection Agency and Lead-Based Paint

The Environmental Protection Agency (EPA) has enacted disclosure requirements to ensure that renters, buyers, lessors, landlords, and property managers are made aware of lead-based paint hazards in housing built prior to 1978. The EPA has also produced consumer protection information, such as the fact sheet shown in exhibit 5.1.

The Manchester Community

Manchester is New Hampshire's largest and most ethnically and racially diverse city. Due in part to its location on the Merrimack River, it has a rich history in textile manufacturing. Representing 10 percent of the state's total population, the city serves as a microcosm exemplifying the societal and economic issues experienced elsewhere.

New Hampshire has some of the oldest housing stock in the United States, with almost 40 percent of rental housing and 28 percent of owner-occupied housing built

EXHIBIT 5.1
Environmental
Protection
Agency Lead
Paint Fact Sheet

United States Environmental Protection Agency	Prevention, Pesticides, and Toxic Substances (7404)	EPA-747-F-96-002 March 1996 (Revised 12/96)

FACT SHEET

EPA and HUD Move to Protect Children from Lead-Based Paint Poisoning; Disclosure of Lead-Based Paint Hazards in Housing

SUMMARY

The Environmental Protection Agency (EPA) and the Department of Housing and Urban Development (HUD) are announcing efforts to ensure that the public receives the information necessary to prevent lead poisoning in homes that may contain lead-based paint hazards. Beginning this fall, most home buyers and renters will receive known information on lead-based paint and lead-based paint hazards during sales and rentals of housing built before 1978. Buyers and renters will receive specific information on lead-based paint in the housing as well as a Federal pamphlet with practical, low-cost tips on identifying and controlling lead-based paint hazards. Sellers, landlords, and their agents will be responsible for providing this information to the buyer or renter before sale or lease.

LEAD-BASED PAINT IN HOUSING

Approximately three-quarters of the nation's housing stock built before 1978 (approximately 64 million dwellings) contains some lead-based paint. When properly maintained and managed, this paint poses little risk. However, 1.7 million children have blood-lead levels above safe limits, mostly due to exposure to lead-based paint hazards.

EFFECTS OF LEAD POISONING

Lead poisoning can cause permanent damage to the brain and many other organs and causes reduced intelligence and behavioral problems. Lead can also cause abnormal fetal development in pregnant women.

BACKGROUND

To protect families from exposure to lead from paint, dust, and soil, Congress passed the Residential Lead-Based Paint Hazard Reduction Act of 1992, also

known as Title X. Section 1018 of this law directed HUD and EPA to require the disclosure of known information on lead-based paint and lead-based paint hazards before the sale or lease of most housing built before 1978.

WHAT IS REQUIRED

Before ratification of a contract for housing sale or lease:

- Sellers and landlords must disclose known lead-based paint and lead-based paint hazards and provide available reports to buyers or renters.

- Sellers and landlords must give buyers and renters the pamphlet, developed by EPA, HUD, and the Consumer Product Safety Commission (CPSC), titled *Protect Your Family from Lead in Your Home*.

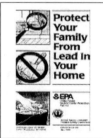

- Home buyers will get a 10-day period to conduct a lead-based paint inspection or risk assessment at their own expense. The rule gives the two parties flexibility to negotiate key terms of the evaluation.

- Sales contracts and leasing agreements must include certain notification and disclosure language.

- Sellers, lessors, and real estate agents share responsibility for ensuring compliance.

(continued)

EXHIBIT 5.1
Environmental
Protection
Agency Lead
Paint Fact Sheet
(continued)

WHAT IS NOT REQUIRED
- This rule does not require any testing or removal of lead-based paint by sellers or landlords.

- This rule does not invalidate leasing and sales contracts.

TYPE OF HOUSING COVERED
Most private housing, public housing, Federally owned housing, and housing receiving Federal assistance are affected by this rule.

TYPE OF HOUSING NOT COVERED
- Housing built after 1977 (Congress chose not to cover post-1977 housing because the CPSC banned the use of lead based paint for residential use in 1978).

- Zero-bedroom units, such as efficiencies, lofts, and dormitories.

- Leases for less than 100 days, such as vacation houses or short-term rentals.

- Housing for the elderly (unless children live there).

- Housing for the handicapped (unless children live there).

- Rental housing that has been inspected by a certified inspector and found to be free of lead-based paint.

- Foreclosure sales.

EFFECTIVE DATES
- For owners of more than 4 dwelling units, the effective date is September 6, 1996.

- For owners of 4 or fewer dwelling units, the effective date is December 6, 1996.

THOSE AFFECTED
The rule will help inform about 9 million renters and 3 million home buyers each year. The estimated cost associated with learning about the requirements, obtaining the pamphlet and other materials, and conducting disclosure activities is about $6 per transaction.

EFFECT ON STATES AND LOCAL GOVERNMENTS
This rule should not impose additional burdens on states since it is a Federally administered and enforced requirement. Some state laws and regulations require the disclosure of lead hazards in housing. The Federal regulations will act as a complement to existing state requirements.

FOR MORE INFORMATION
- For a copy of *Protect Your Family from Lead in Your Home* (in English or Spanish) , the sample disclosure forms, or the rule, call the National Lead Information Clearinghouse (NLIC) at (800) 424–LEAD, or TDD (800) 526–5456 for the hearing impaired. You may also send your request by fax to (202) 659–1192 or by Internet E-mail to ehc@cais.com. Visit the NLIC on the Internet at http://www.nsc.org/nsc/ehc/ehc.html.

- Bulk copies of the pamphlet are available from the Government Printing Office (GPO) at (202) 512–1800. Refer to the complete title or GPO stock number 055–000–00507–9. The price is $26.00 for a pack of 50 copies. Alternatively, persons may reproduce the pamphlet, for use or distribution, if the text and graphics are reproduced in full. Camera-ready copies of the pamphlet are available from the National Lead Information Clearinghouse.

- For specific questions about lead-based paint and lead-based paint hazards, call the National Lead Information Clearinghouse at (800) 424–LEAD, or TDD (800) 526–5456 for the hearing impaired.

- The EPA pamphlet and rule are available electronically and may be accessed through the Internet.
  Electronic Access:
  Gopher: gopher.epa.gov:70/11/Offices/PestPreventToxic/Toxic/lead_pm
  WWW: http://www.epa.gov/opptintr/lead/index.html
  http://www.hud.gov
  Dial up: (919) 558–0335
  FTP: ftp.epa.gov (*To login, type "anonymous." Your password is your Internet E-mail address.*)

Source: Reprinted from Environmental Protection Agency (2018).

prior to 1950. Approximately 77 percent of Manchester's housing units were built prior to bans on lead-based paint, and the housing stock in the center city neighborhoods is generally of poor quality (MHD 2005; New Hampshire Department of Health and Human Services 2016a). These environmental factors contribute to a heightened risk for lead exposure.

Manchester is a designated refugee resettlement community, per the US State Department, and has experienced increasing cultural diversity as a result. This diversity, in turn, requires that the city's public health, healthcare, and community service systems be able to manage individuals from different backgrounds and with varying interpretations of health (MHD 2018; Bazos and Thomas 2008).

Describing Manchester, Caron and Serrell (2009, 197) write: "This community's ecology has created a densely populated and impoverished center city area surrounded by a less populated and more prosperous suburban community."

The Refugee Resettlement Process

The New Hampshire Office of Minority Health and Refugee Affairs oversees the state's refugee resettlement program, working closely with voluntary resettlement agencies and area partners (New Hampshire Department of Health and Human Services 2016b). Once a community is determined to have the capacity to receive refugees, it is given a notice of one to two weeks that refugees are on their way.

The resettlement agency assists with core resettlement services, including orientation to the community's governance, employment opportunities, and healthcare system. Additional core services may involve assisting refugee families with renting and furnishing an apartment; connecting families to food stamps and Medicaid; and registering children for school. The agency may also help adults with registration for English for Speakers of Other Languages classes, which teach not only language but also life skills, such as how to open a bank account or complete an application, as well as parenting support.

The resettlement process focuses on the essential skills needed to live, work, and go to school in Manchester; however, it generally does not address cultural competence beyond that level. Health insurance and the health system are explained, but only superficially. Refugees are not tested for health literacy—for instance, the ability to read a prescription, understand doctors' orders, or use current technology to schedule appointments.

The resettlement agency is the link between the refugee and the community in the early days of the resettlement process. Assistance from the resettlement agency follows a declining model of support, whereby the services provided typically last for four to six months. If further assistance is needed after that period, the refugee must initiate contact with the resettlement agency. The overall measure of a resettlement agency's success is that "a resettled refugee obtains employment" (Caron and Tshabangu-Soko 2012)—not that the refugee has adapted culturally.

Within two weeks of arrival, all refugees resettling in Manchester are seen at the Manchester Health Department for an initial assessment by a community health nurse. The MHD's Refugee Health Program includes the following components (MHD 2018):

- Initial health assessment
- Tuberculin skin testing
- Medical evaluation
- Immunizations
- Lead screenings
- Health orientation classes

Childhood Lead Poisoning as a Wicked Problem

Fatalities from pediatric lead poisoning are rare: The child in Manchester was the first reported lead-poisoning death in the United States since 1990 (Caron et al. 2001). Nonetheless, childhood lead poisoning has been described as a persistent wicked problem, because its dynamic and multifactorial nature can make it resistant to resolution (Caron and Serrell 2009). Young children may be particularly vulnerable to the health effects of lead because of their low body weight and hand-to-mouth activity, and the effects may be worse for children with iron deficiency or poor nutritional status.

Lead is characterized as a neurotoxin that can lead to hyperactivity; impairments in speech, hearing, learning, and memory; and irreversible brain damage. Epidemiologic studies have found an inverse association between children's intellectual functioning and lower blood lead concentrations (CDC 2005), and these findings have prompted the CDC to repeatedly lower its definition of the level of concern. As of 2019, the level was at 5 micrograms of lead per deciliter of blood (5 µg/dL).

Despite the public health advances aimed at removing lead from the environment—specifically from gasoline and paint—exposure to lead remains a persistent hazard in many regions. In 2000, an estimated 434,000 US children had blood lead levels of 10 µg/dL or higher (Agency for Toxic Substances and Disease Registry 2019; CDC 2005).

A significant percentage of the lead-poisoned children in the Manchester Health Department's caseload have been refugees or children of refugees. Many refugees do not speak or read English, and many are unaware of the lead-poisoning risks associated with poor housing and environmental conditions. The CDC recommends that all one- and two-year-old children residing in Manchester be tested for lead paint exposure (MHD 2002).

Community Agencies and Stakeholders

Following the pediatric lead-poisoning fatality in Manchester, an academic–community partnership emerged among existing organizations. The partnership included the MHD, with several decades of experience in case management and education on lead hazards; the Dartmouth Toxic Metals Research Program's Community Outreach Group, a program funded by the National Institute of Environmental Health Sciences; and the Greater Manchester Partners Against Childhood Lead Poisoning, a broad-based community coalition with representatives from low-income housing organizations, educators, a minority health coalition, clinicians, the state Childhood Lead Poisoning Prevention Program, rental property owners, property managers, and parents whose children had been poisoned by lead paint (Caron and Serrell 2009). The partnership worked to develop a quality-improvement screening tool that would help ensure that all children in the Manchester community were screened for lead exposure during their well-child visits.

Development of Public Policy Regarding Prevention and Amelioration

The following historical perspective from the City of Manchester Health Department (2002) chronicles the department's prevention efforts and activities with regard to childhood lead poisoning:

> During the 1970's, lead was removed from paint by federal order. In addition, lead in the air declined markedly as its use as a gasoline additive was substantially reduced. During the 1970's, various preventive initiatives were employed within the City of Manchester. The following summarizes the local historical milestones from 1976 to the present.
>
> - 1976—A system was established whereby the results of all blood lead analyses performed at the State Laboratories were reported to the Manchester Health Department.
> - 1977—The Manchester Health Department (MHD) published the *Estimation of the Extent and Nature of Lead-Paint Poisoning in Manchester, NH.* The report cites that from 1975–1977, 56 children with elevated blood lead levels of at least 40 µg/dl were reported. The report also estimated the number of elevated blood lead levels in children under the age of six from Manchester's twenty-six Census Tracts was between 465 and 521. It was determined that of Manchester's 30,070 housing units (1970 data), 67.2% or 20,333 units were built prior to 1940. When the environmental investigation

(continued)

revealed that lead paint was accessible to children, a letter was sent to the property owner urging that proper measures be implemented to prevent the future occurrence of lead poisonings.

- 1977—Grant funding was sought to increase lead screening efforts and establish a Division of Lead Poisoning Prevention at the MHD.
- 1977—Senate Bill 320 promoted the establishment of a statewide program to prevent lead poisoning.
- 1978—Lead poisoning specialists from the Centers for Disease Control worked with MHD staff to implement a lead screening clinic to identify youngsters with elevated blood lead levels and estimate the extent of childhood lead poisoning within the community.
- 1980—House Bill 788 was passed adopting federal standards to prohibit the use of lead-based substances in dwellings.
- 1987—Lead was removed from plumbing solder.
- 1989—Health Department sanitarians collected 672 samples from bubblers and water coolers in 25 Manchester schools. Testing was performed by laboratory personnel at the Manchester Water Works using EPA-approved methodologies. Of the 672 samples collected, 138 (20%) exceeded the 20 ppb (parts per billion) lead level recommended by EPA. The MHD put forth recommendations that water coolers and bubblers with levels over 20 ppb should be resampled and put out of service until lead levels were reduced to below 20 ppb.
- 1989—The City of Manchester amended its Code of Ordinances to include the provisions of NH RSA-130-A, relative to lead poisoning prevention and control. If a child is determined to have an elevated blood lead level >= 20 µg/dl, the MHD will conduct environmental investigations, issue abatement orders, and enforce such orders. These activities continued through June 30, 1992 through the use of City funds.
- 1992—In July, the State of New Hampshire Childhood Lead Poisoning Prevention Program (NH CLPPP) received funding from the CDC to address childhood lead poisoning prevention throughout the State. NH CLPPP contracted with the MHD to perform environmental investigations, issue abatement orders, and enforce the orders.
- 1992—Following the changes in the federal definition of childhood lead poisoning, the State of New Hampshire reported an increase in lead poisoning cases from 96 in Fiscal Year 1991 to more than 700 in Fiscal Year 1992. The State of NH sought additional funding of $245,600.00 to enhance lead poisoning prevention efforts. The additional funding would permit the State to designate a chief of the lead poisoning prevention program and hire a nurse and an environmentalist.

(continued)

- 1992—The MHD received funding from the State of NH to hire a Public Health Specialist responsible for conducting lead poisoning prevention activities over a five-year period.
- 1993—The MHD hired a part-time (24 hours per week) Community Health Nurse to provide lead case management services.
- 1994—Funding from the NH Department of Health and Human Services provided for an additional Community Health Nurse to provide lead screenings at WIC (Women, Infants and Children) Clinics.
- 1995—The Manchester Health Department published a report on the cost-effectiveness of case management in the *Journal of Environmental Health*.
- 1995—The current RSA 130-A was passed, which provides authority for the State of NH to implement a training, licensure, and regulatory program. The legislation also required the State to conduct surveillance of childhood lead poisoning, provide case management services to children with confirmed elevated blood lead $> = 15$ μg/dl and collaborate with local public health departments, property owners, health care providers and others to provide prevention programs.
- 1996–1997—Additional funding allowed for the expansion of case management services from 24 to 40 hours per week at the MHD.
- 1997—NH CLPPP no longer provided funding for the MHD to conduct environmental investigations and enforcement activities. By State authority, the NH CLPPP assumed the responsibility for these activities in Manchester. It was determined that until the City Ordinance is repealed, the NH CLPPP will conduct inspections, the MHD will issue the abatement order, and the NH CLPPP will assume responsibility for enforcement of said orders. On July 28, 1997 the repeal of Chapter 12 of the City of Manchester Code of Ordinances began. The final reading and incorporation of revised Chapter into Code of Ordinances occurred on October 7, 1997.
- 1997–1998—Funding for lead screenings at Manchester WIC Clinics ceased.
- 2001—Funding for case management services at the Manchester Health Department was reduced. As of July 1, 2001, the nurse case manager was funded to provide 24 hours per week of case management services again.
- March 2002—The MHD began the provision of lead screenings one-day per week at WIC Clinics.

Contemporary Concerns and Next Steps

The pediatric lead-poisoning fatality described in this case attracted widespread attention and prompted efforts at various levels to address the problem (including a New Hampshire state law passed in 2018). Nonetheless, the problem persists, both in Manchester and throughout the nation.

The community leaders of Manchester's academic–community partnership now wonder how they should update their activities to reflect changing knowledge about lead poisoning; cultural sensitivity, particularly with regard to the continuing influx of immigrant populations; public and professionals' awareness of lead-poisoning risks; data systems that convey clinical and social information; and state and federal regulations.

Questions

Fact and Data Analysis Questions

1. Describe the demographics of the City of Manchester, New Hampshire. What secondary data sets might be used to study these demographics, thereby avoiding the costs of collecting primary data?
2. What is cultural competence? Why is this concept relevant to the problem in New Hampshire?
3. What is health literacy? How might it be relevant to this case?
4. Explain how the community environment contributes to the childhood lead-poisoning problem.
5. What about the availability of data might contribute to the difficulty of recognizing and correctly diagnosing a patient's condition as lead poisoning?
6. What are "acceptable" levels of lead in community dwellings? How and why have the standards changed over time?
7. If a health center knew that its community had high prevalence of an unusual condition and wanted to add information about the condition to its electronic health record (EHR), what would be the process for gathering and storing data not programmed into standard EHRs?

Discussion Questions

1. Analyze the multisector systems involved in childhood lead poisoning.
2. Apply the Ecological Model of Health to childhood lead poisoning.
3. Identify and critique the roles and responsibilities of the various stakeholders, and postulate a model for anchor and backbone institutions to use in identification, prevention, diagnosis, and treatment of lead poisoning.

4. Who (i.e., what component of the community's healthcare system) is responsible for addressing this persistent public health problem? Who else should be involved, and why?

5. Postulate how the child in this case encountered the lead-paint risk and how the community could be affected by such a tragedy.

6. Develop a prevention approach for childhood lead poisoning in urban communities similar to Manchester, New Hampshire.

7. How would you measure the effectiveness of the childhood lead-poisoning prevention approach you designed? Describe the variables you would use.

8. Explain the role of cultural competence and health literacy in this persistent public health issue. How might education be provided, and to whom, to help address these two concerns?

9. If you were designing a tool to help primary care clinics screen for social determinants of health, what would you include? What metrics would you use? How would you use the information gained?

10. What could be done to educate or guide clinicians about lead poisoning that would increase their awareness and their likelihood of diagnosing the condition?

11. In tracing the regulatory history of lead-poisoning control efforts, who have been the advocates for implementation and for ongoing changes?

12. As the leaders of Manchester's academic–community partnership ponder the future of lead-poisoning prevention, what existing practices should they maintain? What new initiatives should they explore? How will continued demographic change be considered in the evolution of regulations and practice?

References

Agency for Toxic Substances and Disease Registry (ATSDR). 2019. "Toxicological Profile for Lead." Accessed June 6. www.atsdr.cdc.gov/ToxProfiles/tp.asp?id=96&tid=22.

Bazos, D., and A. Thomas. 2008. *Manchester's Primary Care Safety Net "Intact but Endangered": A Call to Action*. City of Manchester Department of Health. Published June 2. www.manchesternh.gov/portals/2/departments/health/a%20call%20to%20action%20-%20 6%202%202008.pdf.

Caron, R. M., R. DiPentima, C. Alvarado, P. Alexakos, J. Filiano, T. Gilson, J. Greenblatt, G. Robinson, N. Twitchell, L. Speikers, M. A. Abdel-Nasser, H. A. El-Henawy, M. Markowitz, and P. Ashley. 2001. "Fatal Pediatric Lead Poisoning—New Hampshire, 2000." *Morbidity and Mortality Weekly Report* 50 (22): 457–59.

Caron, R. M., and N. Serrell. 2009. "Community Ecology and Capacity: Keys to Improving the Environmental Communication of Wicked Problems." *Applied Environmental Education and Communication: An International Journal* 8 (3): 195–203.

Caron, R. M., and T. S. Tshabangu-Soko. 2012. "Environmental Inequality: Childhood Lead Poisoning as an Inadvertent Consequence of the Refugee Resettlement Process." *Journal of Progressive Human Services* 23 (3): 208–22.

Centers for Disease Control and Prevention (CDC). 2019. "Blood Lead Levels in Children." Reviewed July 30. www.cdc.gov/nceh/lead/acclpp/blood_lead_levels.htm.

———. 2005. *Preventing Lead Poisoning in Young Children.* Published August. www.cdc.gov/ nceh/lead/publications/books/plpyc/contents.htm.

City of Manchester Health Department (MHD). 2018. "Refugee Health Program." Accessed August 20. www.manchesternh.gov/Departments/Health/Services/Refugee-Health.

———. 2005. "Archived Health Data: Manchester Health Department 2005 Report Card." Accessed June 6, 2019. www.manchesternh.gov/Departments/Health/Public-Health-Data/ Archived-Health-Data.

———. 2002. *Preventing Childhood Lead Poisoning in Manchester, New Hampshire: Recommendations for the Community.* Published September. www.manchesternh.gov/portals/2/ departments/health/Preventing%20Childhood%20Lead%20Poisoning%20Sept%202002. pdf.

Environmental Protection Agency (EPA). 2018. "Fact Sheet: EPA and HUD Move to Protect Children from Lead-Based Paint Poisoning; Disclosure of Lead-Based Paint Hazards in Housing." Accessed June 6. www.epa.gov/lead/fact-sheet-epa-and-hud-move-protect- children-lead-based-paint-poisoning-disclosure-lead-based.

New Hampshire Department of Health and Human Services. 2016a. "Healthy Homes and Lead Poisoning Prevention Program." Accessed June 27, 2018. www.dhhs.nh.gov/dphs/bchs/ clpp/index.htm.

———. 2016b. "New Hampshire Refugee Program." Accessed June 7, 2019. www.dhhs.nh.gov/ omh/refugee/index.htm.

Useful Resources

- American Community Survey (www.census.gov/programs-surveys/acs/)
- Centers for Disease Control and Prevention—Social Determinants of Health (www.cdc. gov/socialdeterminants/)
- Centers for Medicare & Medicaid Services—*A Practical Guide to Implementing the National CLAS Standards* (https://www.cms.gov/About-CMS/Agency-Information/ OMH/Downloads/CLAS-Toolkit-12-7-16.pdf)
- Environmental Protection Agency—Lead (www.epa.gov/lead)
- Greater Manchester Community Health Needs Assessment (www.elliothospital.org/ website/downloads/QualitativeNeedsAssessment.pdf); built upon the 2014 Manchester Neighborhood Health Improvement Strategy (www.manchesternh.gov/health/ NeighborhoodHealthImprovementStrategy.pdf) and the 2016 Greater Manchester, New Hampshire, Health Improvement Plan (www.manchesternh.gov/Portals/2/ Departments/health/GManCHIP.pdf)

- National Lead Information Center (1-800-424-LEAD)
- National Standards for Culturally and Linguistically Appropriate Services (CLAS) in Health and Health Care (www.thinkculturalhealth.hhs.gov/clas)
- University of Kansas Community Tool Box (https://ctb.ku.edu/en)
- US Department of Housing and Urban Development—Office of Lead Hazard Control and Healthy Homes (www.hud.gov/lead)

PUBLIC HEALTH

Charles-Edward Amory Winslow (1920, 30) famously defined *public health* as "the science and art of preventing disease, prolonging life, and promoting physical health and efficiency through organized community efforts for the sanitation of the environment, the control of community infections, the education of the individual in principles of personal hygiene, the organization of medical and nursing service for the early diagnosis and preventive treatment of disease, and the development of the social machinery which will ensure to every individual in the community a standard of living adequate for the maintenance of health."

Roughly 100 years later, the World Health Organization (WHO), which advances public health initiatives at the global level, continues to use this definition in a simplified form: Public health is "the art and science of preventing disease, prolonging life, and promoting health through the organized efforts of society" (WHO 2019).

Public Health in the United States

In many countries, public health is the core of the national healthcare system. The United States, however, has developed public health as a system separate from the healthcare delivery system. Public and private activities do overlap, but in a way unique to each community.

Government-sponsored public health in the United States has distinct federal, state, and local components:

- At the federal level, the leading entity is the Centers for Disease Control and Prevention (CDC). Information is available at www.cdc.gov.
- Public health at the state level has 50 distinct entities representing the state governments, as well as designated public health units serving US territories and the District of Columbia. Information about state health departments can be accessed through the Association of State and Territorial Health Officials, at www.astho.org.

- Local health departments (LHDs) serve county or city jurisdictions. The National Association of County and City Health Officials (NACCHO) provides information about LHDs at www.naccho.org.
- Tribal health jurisdictions, which are organized under the Indian Health Service (IHS), serve Native Americans and other indigenous groups. Information about the IHS can be found at www.ihs.gov.

Funding for these entities flows from the federal government to the state and local levels. In addition, states and local health departments obtain their own funding from taxes and special assessments, as well as grants and other sources.

Ten Essential Functions

The CDC (2018) has defined Ten Essential Public Health Functions (see exhibit 1), grouped into three major areas, plus one overarching area:

- The "Assessment" area includes the following functions: (1) monitor health and (2) diagnose and investigate.
- The "Policy Development" area includes (3) inform, educate, and empower; (4) mobilize community partnerships; and (5) develop policies.
- "Assurance" includes (6) enforce laws, (7) link to services / provide care, (8) assure competent workforce, and (9) evaluate.
- "System Management," an overarching area, includes the final function: (10) research.

Every public health department in the United States is expected to carry out all ten functions; implementation, however, varies by agency. The role of each public health agency depends on state and local laws, available assets in the community, and the needs of the community the agency serves. Public health agencies make an effort to complement, not duplicate, the services of other organizations in the community.

Public Health Accreditation

Public health agencies were one of the last types of health entities in the United States to be accredited by an independent agency. The Public Health Accreditation Board (PHAB) launched the first national accreditation program for public health departments in 2011 (Robert Wood Johnson Foundation 2011). PHAB accredits local and state health departments based on their performance of all ten essential functions, as

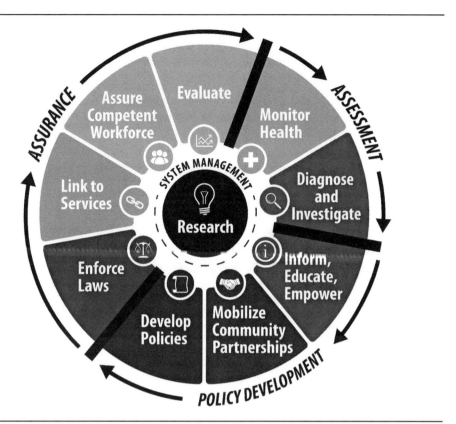

EXHIBIT 1
Ten Essential
Public Health
Services

Source: Reprinted from CDC (2018).

well as on their completion of or participation in a community health needs assessment. The purpose of accreditation is to ensure a basic level of performance for each agency and to promote standardization across locations. Accreditation standards are publicly available and can be accessed at www.phaboard.org.

Public Health in Other Sectors

Public health functions are also performed by myriad other organizations, including nonprofit, for-profit, and public entities. For example, health systems, insurance companies, pharmaceutical companies, and universities are all frequent contributors to public health initiatives. Other government agencies, such as Area Agencies on Aging, Federally Qualified Health Centers, and mental health clinics, also engage in public health activities. The total funding and human resources devoted to these efforts are difficult to calculate. Local and state governmental public health departments may assume the role of convener, coordinator, or information repository.

Cases

The cases in this section of the book explore public health issues from different perspectives. Case 6 examines how programs and structures at the state level affect local public health activities carried out by public and private organizations, whereas case 7 looks at how a local public health department brings together entities in the community to collaborate on projects pertaining to a topic of common interest.

References

Centers for Disease Control and Prevention (CDC). 2018. "The Public Health System & the 10 Essential Public Health Services." Reviewed June 26. www.cdc.gov/publichealthgateway/publichealthservices/essentialhealthservices.html.

Robert Wood Johnson Foundation. 2011. "Public Health Accreditation Board Launches National Accreditation for Health Departments." Published September 14. www.rwjf.org/en/library/articles-and-news/2011/09/public-health-accreditation-board-launches-national-accreditatio.html.

Winslow, C.-E. A. 1920. "The Untilled Fields of Public Health." *Science* 51 (1306): 23–33.

World Health Organization (WHO). 2019. "Public Health Services." Accessed June 11. www.euro.who.int/en/health-topics/Health-systems/public-health-services.

GOVERNANCE AND POWER SHARING: BUILDING COMMUNITY PARTNERSHIPS FOR POPULATION HEALTH GAINS IN RURAL MINNESOTA

James A. Rice

Note: This case is based on a composite of real experiences and includes details added for pedagogical purposes. The personal names are fictitious. Countryside Public Health has given permission for the use of its name.

Case at a Glance

Overarching themes The themes of this case are (1) the structure and funding of public health in the United States and (2) the collaboration of public and private agencies to address health issues facing the community.

Learning objectives
- Evaluate the structure of the US public health system, including the federal, state, and local facets.
- Describe the funding streams for public health programs in the United States.
- Differentiate public/population health from individual health approaches to health problems.
- Characterize the residents of rural areas, and assess their health characteristics.
- Contrast health systems in rural areas with those in urban/metropolitan areas.
- Analyze the power structure of a community.
- Articulate a multisector, cross-boundary approach to addressing a public health problem, with measurable outcomes.
- Identify sources of evidence about the effectiveness of health interventions and health promotion programs.
- Develop a community health improvement plan.
- Describe the opioid epidemic and approaches to resolution.

Key terms
- Collective impact
- Critical access hospital
- Local health department (LHD)
- Opioid epidemic
- Public health

	• Sources of power • State health department (SHD)
Management competencies	Planning a community health improvement plan, managing collaboration among organizations
Population/ subgroup	Residents of rural areas
Health issue or condition	Opioid epidemic

Management Challenge

Clas Johnsson is the executive director of the Chippewa County Health Department in Minnesota. Currently, he is also serving a three-year rotating term as head of Countryside Public Health (CPH). CPH is a collaborative agency of partners throughout five rural Minnesota counties: Big Stone, Chippewa, Lac qui Parle, Swift, and Yellow Medicine (CPH 2019a). During his term, Clas is responsible for guiding CPH's strategic plan and preparing the annual community health improvement plan (CHIP). This year's CHIP will be different from those of previous years because of the opioid epidemic that has been sweeping through Minnesota. Clas needs to figure out how to address the opioid epidemic while still sustaining attention to the area's chronic health challenges, such as obesity.

Background

The counties of this rural area of Minnesota are working collectively under the infrastructure for public health established by the state. Under this infrastructure, various organizations come together to develop and govern diverse community health partnerships to achieve sustainable health gains. The organizations participating in a partnership start by developing a shared long-term vision for health and then create a joint CHIP.

Public Health in Minnesota

Minnesota's public health system is a state and local partnership known as the Community Health Services (CHS) system. It was created by the Community Health Services Act (Minn. Stat. § 145A), an innovative state law that was passed in 1976 and subsequently revised in 1987 and 2003. Now called the Local Public Health Act, the legislation delineates the responsibilities of the state (via the Minnesota Department of Health), city, and county governments in the planning, development, funding, and delivery of public health services (Minnesota Department of Health 2017).

The CHS system provides the infrastructure for nearly all public health efforts in Minnesota, and it enables state and local governments to combine resources to serve

Key Acronyms and Initials

This case uses numerous acronyms and initials, a number of which are similar. The following list is provided to help minimze confusion:

- **CHIP**: community health improvement plan (a plan created by a community health partnership to comply with Minnesota's state mandates)
- **CHS**: Community Health Services system (a collaboration of counties reporting to the state)
- **CPH**: Countryside Public Health (a specific community health partnership serving five counties in Minnesota)
- **SHIP**: State Health Improvement Plan or Statewide Health Improvement Partnership (a coordinated strategy that sets out priorities for local partnerships to incorporate into their CHIPs)

public health needs in a more efficient, cost-effective way. The system is structured to be flexible, so it can meet the various needs of communities throughout the state and promote direct and timely communications between state and local health departments. The CHS system relies on shared goals among community agencies and a desire to work together to improve the lives of all Minnesotans (see exhibit 6.1).

Minnesota's state-level initiatives are formulated into the State Health Improvement Plan (SHIP), which promotes public health intiatives in schools, workplaces, healthcare organizations, and communities. SHIP is working to expand the opportunities for active living, healthy eating, breastfeeding support, and tobacco-free living, as well as address the growing opioid epidemic. In addition, special efforts must be made to meet the needs of growing Hispanic and Asian Pacific population segments.

Collaborative governance through sustainable community health partnerships presents significant opportunities, but it is not easy. Effective collaboration requires

---

EXHIBIT 6.1
Blueprint for Healthy Communities in Minnesota

- Build capacity of local leaders, organizations, and health departments to promote health.
- Research communities' exposure to environmental hazards, local disease prevalence, and more.
- Advocate for policies that improve the health of local community environments.
- Develop partnerships across sectors to advance policy and environmental change strategies to improve health and equity outcomes.

Source: Minnesota Department of Health (2010).

unique leadership players, processes, and systems, as well as significant human and financial resources. Methods must be developed to ensure that interorganizational planning is data driven, open to new wisdom about social determinants of health, and properly coordinated around the framework of collective impact.

Collective impact is a relatively new concept applied to community-wide health-care challenges. It posits that organizations can accomplish more by working together than by working individually, and it is more structured and focused than informal collaboration. A formal model of collective impact lists a number of key concepts and principles of practice, including an emphasis on communication, cross-sector partnerships, mutually reinforcing activities, and measurable outcomes (Collective Impact Forum 2019).

None of Minnesota's public health agencies can meet its mandate alone. Each needs new partners and resources to make sustainable gains in population health.

Challenges to Rural Areas

The pressures on Minnesota's public health system are particularly unrelenting in rural areas. The demographics of such areas are changing, the economy is fragile, and poverty affects many families and children. The financing of healthcare is challenged by a mix of Medicare and Medicaid clients, and health professionals of all disciplines are in short supply. The nationwide opioid epidemic adds to an already extensive list of rural Minnesota's health concerns (see exhibit 6.2).

The Opioid Crisis

The impact of the opioid crisis in Minnesota received widespread attention with the 2016 death of Minnesota-based rock star Prince. He died from a counterfeit prescription drug containing the synthetic opioid fentanyl, and law enforcement officials subsequently acknowledged that such drugs remain far too readily available in Minnesota communities (Magan 2018).

EXHIBIT 6.2
Significant Rural
Health Issues

- The aging population
- Preponderance of chronic conditions
- Access to behavioral health and dental care
- Opioid abuse and treatment
- Healthcare workforce shortages/development
- Nonemergency medical transportation
- Demographic change / growing ethnic diversity
- Rural health insurance market changes
- Reimbursement disparities
- High proportion of Medicare
- Hospitals, clinics, and nursing homes in crisis
- Social determinants of health
- Broadband shortages and telemedicine
- Poverty rates, especially for children and seniors
- Economy based on farming, with little diversification

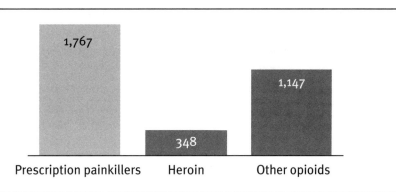

EXHIBIT 6.3
Opioid Deaths in Minnesota

Source: Adapted from Collins (2016); data from the Centers for Disease Control and Prevention.

While detailing a new collaborative to fight the opioid epidemic, one county sheriff commented on the devastating impact of fentanyl: "It's an incredibly insidious chemical that is being introduced into other drugs. . . . This is something that is extremely lethal. It's a very serious problem" (Magan 2018).

Prescription opioids approved by the US Food and Drug Administration have nearly the same chemical composition as illegal heroin (Collins 2016). They are extremely addictive and highly dangerous. Exhibit 6.3 provides a comparison of overdose deaths in Minnesota from prescription painkillers, heroin, and other opioids.

Countryside Public Health and Its Leadership Agencies

Clas Johnsson and Jack Jones are the primary leaders of Countryside Public Health, the CHS agency serving five rural counties in west-central Minnesota. CPH's offices are in Ortonville, Montevideo, Madison, Benson, and Granite Falls. Clas represents the Chippewa County Health Department, and Jack represents a community hospital in Montevideo.

Chippewa County

Chippewa County is in the southwestern region of the state of Minnesota. Its population in the last US census was 12,441 (US Census Bureau 2018). Formed in 1862 and organized in 1868, the county remains focused on farming-related employment and economic development.

The city Montevideo, the county seat of Chippewa County, sits at the intersection of the Minnesota and Chippewa rivers and is surrounded by several smaller communities. A "progressive community with rural values and an evolving economy" (Montevideo Area Chamber of Commerce 2019), Montevideo has been a crossroads for commerce and community building for 250 years. In 2004, the National Civic League named Montevideo an All-America City (National Civic League 2019). Only ten cities per year receive this honor, which is the nation's longest-running and most prestigious civic recognition award.

Though proud of their many assets, the leaders of Montevideo and Chippewa County acknowledge that much work remains to be done to strengthen the community. A top priority is to pursue a bolder set of initiatives for the health of the county's various populations, regardless of age or employment status. Chippewa County is currently experiencing flat population growth, but the composition is changing. The percentages of older adults and people of color are increasing.

The county has an active chamber of commerce and growing civic leadership interest in updating its community health needs assessments and fostering collaboration to establish, implement, and sustain programs and investments for improvements in health. The chamber posts current initiatives and planning processes on its website, so that everyone in the community can be well informed and have an opportunity to participate.

The Community Hospital

Chippewa County–Montevideo Hospital (CCMH), located in Montevideo, is the community hospital that serves the local area. Originally a county hospital supported by local government, it evolved into a 501(c)(3) nonprofit entity that receives a majority of its funding from third-party insurers. The CCMH is a critical access hospital with a seven-person board, half appointed by the county commissioners and half by the city council. Jack Jones has been the hospital's administrator for the past ten years.

Since the previous summer, the CCMH has seen inpatient volume either remain stable or decrease from month to month, which might be good for patients but is not good for the hospital's finances (Gustavo 2014). Medical advancements, both technological and pharmaceutical, have offered "significantly better" care options for patients, according to Jones. However, less volume equals less profit.

According to Jones, managing a healthcare organization in today's rapidly changing environment requires malleability, fortitude, and the ability to constantly adapt. In a sense, Jones must act as a quarterback would if the referee arbitrarily changed the rules of football from one play to the next (Gustavo 2014).

Over many informal lunches, Clas and Jack have discussed French and Raven's (1959) framework for the sources of power, and they have tried to determine who has the greatest power for any given community issue. Multi-agency meetings can be effective for sharing information across sectors, but success will ultimately require concrete actions with specific measures and transparent reporting. A number of boards and board members are actively involved in advancing the community's well-being, but the best collaborative approach for achieving sustainable gains in health status is yet to be determined.

Countryside's Efforts to Mobilize Community Health Partners

Countryside Public Health has prepared its strategic plan for 2013–2018 (Auch 2015), and survey data on the health conditions of each county's residents is available in the *Data Book for Countryside Public Health* (Bartholomay and MartinRogers 2015).

The CPH Community Health Board, headed by Clas, meets at the Chippewa County Family Services Board Room in Montevideo on the second Wednesday of each month. The board's members include a county commissioner from each of the five counties and at-large members primarily from the health field. The relative power of these county commissioners is unequal and may influence how plans are developed and implemented.

CPH is struggling to meet goals of the Statewide Health Improvement Partnership (SHIP). The focus of SHIP is to prevent chronic disease by strengthening the capacity of communities to create their own healthy futures in places where people live, work, learn, and play (CPH 2019b).

CPH would like to take advantage of the funding offered by SHIP, but the agency needs to formulate a plan for doing so. CPH's leaders need to determine how best to implement collaborative program planning for the next three to five years. Moreover, if CPH has any hope of receiving funding through the state's new initiative to address the opioid epidemic, it needs to prepare the annual CHIP with the opioid crisis as the top priority.

Collaboration for sustainable health gains is never easy in rural areas, and the communities served by CPH face a number of challenges as they pursue healthcare's Triple Aim of better population health, better experience of care, and lower per capita cost (Institute for Healthcare Improvement 2019). Civic, business, health, and community leaders have decided to mobilize a diverse "Healthy Community Collaborative" to further define the scope of key health issues and to determine how those issues can be addressed in the most cost-effective manner.

Montevideo and Chippewa County community leaders are particularly interested in the collective impact movement, which has researched various ways to map, plan, and guide community groups. They would like to know how the collective impact approach could help them establish, fund, and govern joint initiatives for health gains.

Community leaders need to collaborate to design and implement the CHIP according to state guidelines. The CHIP should be connected with the strategic plan and consistent with the SHIP, and it should be used to guide a "governing body" of community leaders to improve the health of the population within its jurisdiction. Government agencies—including those related to health, human services, and education—are to use the CHIP collaboratively with community partners to set priorities, coordinate policies and actions, and target resources. A similarly broad, community-level partnership needs to be established to conduct a community health needs assessment (CHNA) to guide the CHIP.

Building Collaborative Governance and Joint Partner Planning

Clas and Jack are meeting to discuss the long-term vision of the CPH strategic plan and the immediate need for the CHIP. Although Clas is the agency's executive director, Jack wields considerable power: He is the head of the five-county region's only critical access hospital and the person who controls the hospital's resources on behalf of its board. Clas and Jack know that, by working together, they can further the missions of their respective organizations.

The CPH governing body needs to have a clear charge or charter document to guide its work. It must ensure that all partners are fully engaged and feel that their needs are being recognized. A critical distinction to make is that the CHIP is *the community's plan for public health*, not public health's plan for the community. The plan must have clear goals and standards, concrete measures, and specific time frames.

Clas and Jack first consider who should be invited to join the advisory board responsible for preparing the CHIP. Potential members include the following:

- County health system administrator/director
- County health system department directors
- County health system supervisors
- Key public health staff
- Hospital or primary care partners
- Community-based organizations
- Schools
- Other county agencies (e.g., social services, public safety, environment)
- Community members
- Businesses
- Foundations
- Representatives of distinct subpopulations (e.g., racial/ethnic groups, age groups, people with disabilities)

Clas and Jack ponder several questions:

- In addition to the CPH board, the Chippewa County Health Department advisory committee, and the hospital's board, do they really need yet *another* board or advisory committee to ensure representation of the community? Should this group be considered a "task force" rather than a "board"? Does the title matter?
- How they will recruit, orient, develop, and support governance decision making by such a diverse group? How can they balance representation of multiple entities with the power of individual leaders?
- What process of collaboration should they recommend to design, establish, and develop the CHIP, and then to ensure ongoing implementation of the CHIP?
- What messages and methods of communication should be sent out to the community at large about the process, the plan, and progress to accomplish the plan?
- How can the leaders best celebrate progress to help sustain engagement and support in future community health enhancement planning work?

Although Minnesota's CHS structure has been in place for several decades, the state is now pushing for critical analysis and use of new organizational arrangements drawn from the collective impact model. The state must approve CPH's strategic plan, which will set forth overarching guidelines for three to five years, and its CHIP, which will focus on one- to two-year implementation tactics aimed at specific problems. Developing a new strategic plan would require a deliberate effort with input from various stakeholders. For now, Clas and Jack decide to focus on getting the CHIP prepared and submitted, with the opioid crisis as their top priority for the coming year.

Their task is all the more difficult because no single template exists for what the state requires for the CHIP. Public health agencies and not-for-profit agencies across the nation have developed CHIPs in response to accrediting requirements imposed by the Public Health Accreditation Board and Internal Revenue Service requirements for nonprofit hospitals.

Clas and Jack take out their napkins at lunch. Jack sketches out what he thinks should be in the CHIP. Clas prepares an organizational chart showing the levels of governance above the box with the new "advisory committee" or "task force" to be selected to create the CHIP. They both order another cup of coffee.

Questions

Fact and Data Analysis Questions

1. What are the essential functions performed by a local, multicounty health department?
2. What are the pertinent urban and rural healthcare delivery differences? What is a critical access hospital?
3. What generic elements should be used to frame the CHIP? Prepare the outline for CPH's CHIP.
4. How can CPH identify evidence-based programs to prevent opioid problems in its rural community? What are some sources of evidence-based programs for health promotion?
5. What organizations should be represented in the group developing the CHIP, particularly if the top priority is to address opioid problems?

Discussion Questions

1. Minnesota has a unique structure for its state public health department. Select another state, and compare its structure and funding of public health with Minnesota's.
2. Trace the funding of opioid programs from federal sources through state and local agencies.

3. How, if at all, does the opioid epidemic manifest differently in rural areas as opposed to urban areas?

4. What will be measures of success in curbing opioid use in the five counties represented by CHP?

5. What are the sources of power, according to French and Raven? How can power among community agencies be determined? Measured?

6. How does the collective impact model differ from a traditional model of collaboration?

7. What measures can be used to determine the success of CPH's efforts to address the chronic health problems of the area? Would the success of collective impact be measured differently? How are measures determined and agreed upon by members?

8. What factors influence how collective impact partnerships change over time? How do changes in institutional membership influence the original goals of the collective impact agreement? Do collaborations among community organizations measure their success in similar ways? Assuming the strategic plan for CPH is intended to be for three years, how does it relate to the expectations of a collective impact model?

9. Who should lead the CHIP task force, and how will power and influence be shared?

10. What can be done to prevent members from feeling burned out?

11. Does the CHIP task force include members of the community the plan is trying to support?

12. How does the CPH governing body coordinate work with other community collaboratives? If the state of Minnesota maintains that collaboration through the CHS model is more efficient than individual counties working alone, should collaboration among multiple CHS partnerships be promoted as well? What would be the pros and cons?

13. Once the CHIP has been completed and CPH returns to preparing its next three-year strategic plan, what should be the elements of the planning process? Who should be involved? How will this work differ from the process of preparing the CHIP?

References

Auch, L. 2015. *Countryside Public Health Strategic Plan 2013–2018.* Countryside Public Health. Published January 7. www.countrysidepublichealth.org/newsite/ckfinder/userfiles/files/Countryside%20Public%20Healthstrategicplan.pdf.

Bartholomay, A., and N. MartinRogers. 2015. *Data Book for Countryside Public Health: 2015 Southwest/South Central MN Adult Health Survey.* Countryside Public Health.

Published October. www.countrysidepublichealth.org/ship/ckfinder/userfiles/files/
CountrysideDataBook_Countryside_10-15.pdf.

Collective Impact Forum. 2019. "What Is Collective Impact?" Accessed June 11. www.
collectiveimpactforum.org/what-collective-impact.

Collins, J. 2016. "Here's Why Minnesota Has a Big Problem with Opioid Overdoses."
MPR News. Published April 18. www.mprnews.org/story/2016/04/18/opioid-
overdose-epidemic-explained.

Countryside Public Health (CPH). 2019a. "About Us." Accessed June 12. www.
countrysidepublichealth.org/about.php.

———. 2019b. "Healthy Lifestyles." Accessed June 13. www.countrysidepublichealth.org/
healthy-lifestyles.php.

French, J., and B. Raven. 1959. "The Bases of Social Power." In *Studies in Social Power*, edited by
D. Cartwright, 150–67. Ann Arbor, MI: Institute for Social Research.

Gustavo, S. 2014. "Paulson, CCMH Enduring Changing Finances of Health Care." *Montevideo
American-News*. Published August 28. www.montenews.com/article/20140828/
NEWS/140829563.

Institute for Healthcare Improvement. 2019. "The IHI Triple Aim." Accessed June 13. www.ihi.
org/Engage/Initiatives/TripleAim/Pages/default.aspx.

Magan, C. 2018. "Minnesota's Opioid Crisis Grows More Deadly. Will a New Partnership Address
the Problem?" *Pioneer Press*. Published April 19. www.twincities.com/2018/04/19/
what-are-state-and-local-officials-doing-to-address-the-opioid-crisis/.

Minnesota Department of Health. 2017. "Minnesota Local Public Health Act: Summary of Minn.
Stat. § 145A." Published June. www.health.state.mn.us/communities/practice/lphact/
statute/docs/LPHActSummary.pdf.

———. 2010. *Updating Minnesota's Blueprint for Public Health*. Published December 20.
www.health.state.mn.us/communities/practice/schsac/workgroups/docs/2010-12_f_
updatingblueprint.pdf.

Montevideo Area Chamber of Commerce. 2019. "Economic Development." Accessed June 13.
http://montechamber.com/economic-development/.

National Civic League. 2019. "All-America City Winners." Accessed June 13. www.
nationalcivicleague.org/america-city-award/past-winners/.

US Census Bureau. 2018. "QuickFacts: Chippewa County, Minnesota." Accessed June 12, 2019.
www.census.gov/quickfacts/chippewacountyminnesota.

Useful Resources

- Association of State and Territorial Health Officials (www.astho.org)
- Centers for Disease Control and Prevention (www.cdc.gov)
- County Health Rankings (www.countyhealthrankings.org)
- FSG—How to Lead Collective Impact Working Groups (www.fsg.org/
tools-and-resources/how-to-lead-collective-impact-working-groups)

- Minnesota Department of Health—Community Health Improvement Plan (www.health.state.mn.us/divs/opi/pm/lphap/community/chip.html)
- National Association of County and City Health Officials (www.naccho.org)
- Public Health Accreditation Board (www.phaboard.org)
- Rural Health Information Hub—Critical Access Hospitals (www.ruralhealthinfo.org/topics/critical-access-hospitals)

LOCAL HEALTH DEPARTMENT SPEARHEADS COLLABORATION

Katherine A. Stamatakis, Allese B. McVay, Kristin D. Wilson, Kevin Syberg, Bert Malone, Deborah Markenson, and Eduardo J. Simoes

Case at a Glance

Overarching theme   The overarching theme of this case is how a local public health department mobilizes community organizations to collaborate and address a multicausal, community-wide problem—the obesity epidemic.

Learning objectives
- Describe the ten essential functions of public health as performed by a local health department (LHD).
- Assess how an LHD complies with accreditation criteria, including conducting a community health needs assessment.
- Explain the multiple causes of the obesity epidemic in the United States.
- Apply a logic model to a public health issue.
- Identify successful interventions and best practices for addressing obesity at the population health and community health levels.
- Organize cross-sector collaboration to achieve a multifaceted integration of medical care, public health, and social services to address multicausal problems.
- Analyze the characteristics of cross-sector collaborations between healthcare and public health organizations.
- Evaluate tools to measure and assess the effectiveness of cross-sector collaboration.

Key terms
- Backbone institution
- Collaboration
- Local health department (LHD)
- Logic model
- Obesity
- Public health
- Public Health Accreditation Board (PHAB)
- Stakeholders
- Ten essential functions of public health

Management competencies	Organizing multisector collaboration and measuring success
Population/ subgroup	County residents
Health issue or condition	Obesity

Management Challenge

Charlie Broz is head of the public health department of the city of Centennial, and Kris Hayworth is chief executive officer of Centennial Health Care Hospital (CHCH), the city's largest not-for-profit hospital. Charlie has invited Kris to brainstorm how the Centennial Health Department and CHCH might work together to combat obesity in the community.

With the systemic changes in the US healthcare environment since 2010, effective prevention and treatment of chronic conditions have become critical for a health system's survival. Kris tells Charlie that CHCH has experienced challenges delivering effective and efficient healthcare as the rate of obesity-related conditions and complications in its patient population has increased. Charlie and Kris also discuss the root causes of obesity, such as having easy access to the wrong foods, lacking opportunities to incorporate physical activity into daily lifestyles, and taking a path toward a life of disease. Charlie knew from previous experience working with Kris that CHCH had a broad perspective on the role of healthcare in promoting the health and well-being of children, families, and the community.

Charlie and Kris realize they can only control the policies and programs of their own organizations, but they agree to share information and ideas and look into the development of joint initiatives to address population obesity in Centennial. Between the two of them, Charlie and Kris might come up with one or more initiatives that could make a difference over time.

The management challenge Charlie and Kris face is to develop a plan for community-wide collaboration to reduce obesity, with sufficient detail and likelihood for success to ensure that their respective boards will agree to support the endeavor.

Background

Given that obesity prevalence is 30 percent or higher in more than two-thirds of US counties (reaching as high as 47 percent), community-based and locally oriented obesity prevention and control efforts are a necessity (County Health Rankings & Roadmaps 2016). The implementation challenge may be greater at the local level than at the state level given the large degree of variability in funding structures, areas of programmatic focus, and capacity among local health departments (LHD) and other health-related organizations in the community. Research suggests that LHDs may lack capacity to address obesity prevention in some of the highest burdened communities (Stamatakis et al. 2012) and that finding new opportunities to enhance capacity through strategic linkages with healthcare and other sectors, such as schools, offers promise (National Association of County and City Health Officials 2015; Dietz et al. 2015). A single entity acting alone is unlikely to solve or even diminish the problem.

Personal Perspective

Yvonne is an 11-year old patient at the Centennial City Community Clinic, a Federally Qualified Health Center (FQHC). During her most recent doctor visit, the clinical nurse measured her weight at 200 pounds and her height at 5 feet 7 inches; records indicate she has gained weight since her previous visit. A measure of Yvonne's body mass index classifies her in the obese category. Children in this clinical classification are more likely to develop serious health problems such as type 2 diabetes and heart disease at some point in their lives. Because of her obesity, Yvonne has difficulty participating in many activities, both in school and around the neighborhood, that are typical for children of her age.

Yvonne's parents are also obese. One parent already has type 2 diabetes, and both parents have a higher-than-average risk of developing conditions that will reduce their quality of life, affect their ability to work, lead to expensive medical care, or even lead to death.

Yvonne and her parents live in a low-income community of Centennial. In the last community health needs assessment, the local public health department classified this community as a "food desert" with "little opportunity for leisure time activity," as perceived by community members. Yvonne's parents are wondering how to change their lifestyle to promote better health for the whole family, but they need additional resources and guidance—they aren't sure where to turn.

Over the past decade, regulatory changes have created new opportunities for cross-sector collaboration around obesity prevention. The passage of the Affordable Care Act (ACA) in 2010 provided a legal foundation for widespread reform of the healthcare system around such goals as expanding health insurance coverage, strengthening primary care access, incentivizing prevention, and increasing integration between public health and healthcare (Rosenbaum 2011; Institute of Medicine 2012). Requirements for nonprofit hospitals to conduct periodic community health needs assessments (CHNAs), to engage public health partners in community health planning, and to report their contributions to their communities all contribute to an environment conducive to collaboration.

The CHNA, in particular, serves an important role in bringing the healthcare and public health sectors together for a joint conversation about community needs and health priorities. Joint CHNAs also provide an opportunity to expand cross-sector collaborations on concrete projects.

A Logic Model for Obesity

Charlie and Kris have developed a list of programs and initiatives related to food, nutrition, and physical activity, as well as a list of stakeholders—people and organizations that care about the health of the community or, from a business perspective, have been engaged in activities related to food, nutrition, and physical activity (e.g., companies providing food services to the school district). In addition, they have prepared a logic model showing the factors related to childhood obesity; researched compelling statistics for a 25-second "elevator speech"; and compiled a list of federal, state, and local programs and policy and environmental changes related to childhood obesity, organized according to the ten essential functions of public health (see Centers for Disease Control and Prevention [CDC] 2018).

Charlie and Kris have developed the logic model to show the relationships of the many factors that can contribute to or ameliorate obesity in children and adults. The model's graphic display will be a useful tool to persuade community groups and organizations to be part of the multifaceted program. It will also help the two of them determine which community partners to include in an obesity prevention program.

In their initial discussion, Charlie and Kris brainstormed ways in which various community entities could affect the childhood obesity problem. After creating a rather long but disorganized list, Charlie suggested that they expand the logic model to indicate which types of organizations could intervene in what ways. He further suggested that they could create an example for other institutions by showing how an LHD could focus on obesity through each of the ten essential functions of public health (CDC 2018). For example, to address the function of developing a strong workforce, the LHD could secure access to free online educational programs about obesity and school wellness policies for teachers, LHD staff, and clinical staff of CHCH and physicians' offices.

At some point, Charlie will need to share the local plan with the state health department, which is a source of funds and the overarching governing body for all LHDs in the state. Charlie also would like to get this effort underway quickly so that he can include it in his application for accreditation by the Public Health Accreditation Board (PHAB), to demonstrate how Centennial Health Department mobilizes local entities to share ownership of community-wide problems and their solutions.

Charlie and Kris have convened a focus group of representatives from key stakeholder organizations and members of the community, with the purpose of presenting an overview of the obesity challenge and gathering community input. They engaged group members to contribute their own ideas, thereby generating excitement and increasing the members' willingness to take ownership for future interventions.

The focus group suggested a variety of ways that the organizations could work together:

- By sharing data and methods for conducting CHNAs, which may lead to greater prioritization of obesity prevention
- Through referrals for weight-loss programs
- By encouraging healthcare practitioners to be advocates for local policies
- By ensuring orientation of efforts toward vulnerable and underserved populations

Health Plan Programs to Prevent Obesity

Research shows that healthcare intervention alone cannot drive obesity-related behavioral change; additional community action is needed for impact at the population level (Obesity Society 2010; Office of the Surgeon General 2010; American Academy of Pediatrics Council on Sports Medicine and Fitness and Council on School Health 2006).

A number of health plans have begun using innovative collaborative strategies for overweight prevention among children and adolescents (Dietz et al. 2007; Boyle et al. 2009). These plans find themselves in a critical position to work across sectors to impact both practice and policy, engaging in multidimensional approaches that change both environmental contexts and the medical system through stronger linkages between clinics and community services.

Innovative cross-sector collaborations with local partners such as health departments, schools, employers, and community organizations can enable health plans to exert meaningful influence on policies and environments well outside of the clinic. For instance, school- and community-based initiatives can promote healthy diets and physical activity through media campaigns, public policy changes, and sustainable environmental modification.

A Measurement Challenge

For any program to be sustained over time, success must be documented. Healthcare executives, CEOs of community agencies, directors of health departments, community leaders, and board members all need to know that the resources they invest in a given program are being used wisely to accomplish the intended goals.

For a program addressing childhood obesity, the aim is to prevent children from becoming obese and thereby minimize the chronic conditions related to obesity that might affect those children later in life. Determining the effects of such an intervention will require years of careful tracking, and Charlie and Kris are well aware that they will likely be retired for many years before the results of their collaboration are truly known. In the meantime, however, they need ways to measure and report indications of success to keep the program staff energized, the community partners involved, and the budgets funded.

Charlie and Kris can look to position their program favorably through two types of measurement approaches: (1) by selecting intervention programs based on evidence of success and (2) by measuring the effectiveness of collaboration among stakeholder organizations. If both of these dimensions can be measured and reported regularly, their program will have better likelihood of success and continuation.

Charlie and Kris start by identifying programs that have been effective in the past with children similar to those in their local school district. Useful information is available through both the federal government and private sources, which have compiled and evaluated studies about the effectiveness of obesity interventions for childhood populations. In addition, Charlie and Kris gather and evaluate measures to assess the success of cross-sector collaborations for obesity prevention. Although the CHNAs of recent years have seen collaboration among public health, healthcare, and community agencies to identify needs, little evidence exists that collaboration has continued and been transformed into actions.

Charlie and Kris will need to incorporate outcomes data about children's and adults' weight and the organizational performance of the collaboration into the program's initial goals and SMART objectives (i.e., objectives that are specific, measurable, attainable, relevant, and time bound); these elements should be fully shared with stakeholders and the community.

Evidence-Based Obesity Prevention Programs

Evidence-based obesity prevention programs include interventions that address policy, built environment, and education for healthy eating and physical activity (see exhibit 7.1). Useful sources of information include *The Guide to Community Preventive Services* (Community Guide 2019), a CDC report on "Recommended Community Strategies and Measurements to Prevent Obesity in the United States" (Khan et al. 2009), the Institute of Medicine and National Research Council's (2009) *Local Government Actions to Prevent Childhood Obesity*, the CDC's (2019) Community Health Improvement Navigator database, the Conduent Healthy Communities Institute's (2019) Promising Practices database, and published reviews of interventions for children and adolescents (Yoshida and Simoes 2018).

Kris has been particularly interested in programs implemented by healthcare organizations (hospitals, clinics, and similar facilities, as well as insurance companies) to promote healthy environments for patients as well as visitors and staff. He identified such programs using a list of evidence-based obesity prevention recommendations from the Harvard T.H. Chan School of Public Health (2019).

Community-Based Approaches in Public Health and Community Settings	**EXHIBIT 7.1** Evidence- Based Practices in Obesity Prevention, by Sector

Policies and/or Changes to the Built Environment
- Improve access to healthy food choices in neighborhoods, restaurants, or food retailers.
- Regulate access to unhealthy foods (e.g., tax drinks containing sugar).
- Improve healthy food choices in schools, worksites, or other local facilities.
- Improve healthy food choices through nutrition assistance programs.
- Increase opportunities for physical activity (e.g., "complete streets," bike lanes).
- Encourage physical activity in communities, schools, or work sites.

Educational Interventions
- Provide health education to increase healthy food choices through community-wide efforts or outreach to children/families.
- Conduct health education interventions through community-wide efforts to increase physical activity.
- Launch health education interventions to increase physical activity in schools, work sites, or other local facilities.

Healthcare Provider–Based Interventions
- Have pediatric healthcare providers monitor weight, conduct behavior counseling (regarding healthy eating, sugar-sweetened beverages, physical activity, screen time, etc.), and establish appropriate follow-up procedures and clinic policies.
- Have adult medicine and primary care providers monitor weight, prescribe appropriate follow-up strategies for overweight patients, and design settings to avoid stigmatizing overweight patients.
- Have pre- and postnatal care providers conduct healthy weight counseling, recommend and provide support for breastfeeding, counsel smoking cessation, and screen for gestational diabetes.

Healthcare Providers, Hospitals, and Insurers Bridging Healthcare and Community Prevention
- Have healthcare professionals advocate as leaders and role models to encourage changes in physical activity and nutrition; act across levels (e.g., practice settings, professional organizations, local, state, federal) for policy and built-environment changes; and encourage parents to become advocates in their schools and communities.
- Have hospitals offer healthy food and beverages to patients, visitors, and employees; encourage providers and employees to model healthy eating; and promote breastfeeding among patient and employee new mothers.
- Provide healthcare professional training that includes obesity prevention and lifestyle counseling, have associations distribute position statements and other evidence-based information about obesity prevention, and encourage members to be role models for healthy eating and physical activity.
- Ensure that health insurance providers cover obesity-related services, provide subscribers incentives for maintaining healthy body weight and adopting healthy behaviors, measure and track progress in body mass index through HEDIS data collection, and fund obesity-prevention efforts and participate in community obesity-prevention coalitions.

Note: HEDIS = Healthcare Effectiveness Data and Information Set.

Measures of Collaboration

Charlie and Kris have encountered some difficulty in identifying measures of collaboration that can be used to create the structure and processes for a collaborative project and mark progress toward success. Nonetheless, they have found three measures of collaboration that are evidence based and would work with the organizations in their community.

Measure 1: Levels of Collaboration

After conducting a literature review to look for existing measures and theoretical frameworks that present levels of partnership on a continuum, Charlie and Kris choose the Frey framework (Frey et al. 2006). This framework describes a continuum of partnership that begins with networking; includes the intermediate levels of cooperation, coordination, and coalition; and ends with collaboration (see exhibit 7.2).

Although the Frey framework initially seemed overly academic for two executives who would still be engaged in day-to-day operations, Charlie and Kris thought the approach could help them examine how an organization's level on the partnership continuum influenced the activities it implemented toward obesity prevention. By doing so, they could be more realistic in promoting activities that were feasible within the context of the group dynamics and resource commitment.

Measure 2: Partnership Trust

The trust among community agencies involved in the obesity prevention collaboration will be of prime importance. The organizations that Kris and Charlie would work with—or not work with—have a history of being independent or even competitive, in part as a result of their competition for grants from the local Community Foundation. Cooperation had been minimal, and collaboration nonexistent. Thus, Charlie and Kris know they will need to work hard to explain the importance of collaboration and to

EXHIBIT 7.2
Levels of
Collaboration

Networking	Cooperation	Coordination	Coalition	Collaboration
Awareness of organization	Information provided to each other	Shared information	Shared ideas	Members belonging to one system
Loosely defined roles	Somewhat defined roles	Defined roles	Shared resources	Frequent communication characterized by mutual trust
Little communication	Formal communication	Frequent communication	Frequent and prioritized communication	
All decisions made independently	All decisions made independently	Some shared decision making	Decision making in which all members have a vote	Consensus reached on decisions

Source: Adapted from Frey, Lohmeier, and Tollefson (2006).

Partnership Trust Items
Accessible
Dependable
Good/clear communication
Mutual benefit
Openness/flexibility
Provides accurate information
Relationship building
Responsible
Shares power/responsibilities
Supportive
Truthful
Values differences

EXHIBIT 7.3
Components
of Partnership
Trust

Source: White-Cooper et al. (2009).

create trust among the potential partners. They reason that, if they are transparent about the need for trust and even develop a way to measure it, they will be able to build confidence among the stakeholder organizations—and also among those organizations' own stakeholders, leaders, boards, and people served.

Charlie and Kris have found a partnership trust tool that was developed by a CDC Prevention Research Center and that had been previously research tested (White-Cooper et al. 2009). Its components are shown in exhibit 7.3. The tool asks each participant to rate how often a certain trait occurs in the partnership as a whole (for all partners), and it includes scales for importance of each trait. Charlie and Kris feel that, if all partner organizations were to rate their level of trust each quarter, the collaborative would have an objective measure for identifying problems as they arose.

Measure 3: Community Context

The third measure selected is an adaptation of the Wilder Collaboration Factors Inventory, which captures contextual characteristics around collaboration and the community (Amherst H. Wilder Foundation 2019). As the measures of this tool have been studied and documented, several characteristics have been shown to have the highest importance: (1) recognition that the task would be difficult for a single organization to accomplish alone, (2) leaders' possession of skills conducive to collaborating, (3) inclusion of appropriate stakeholders in the collaboration, (4) a history of agencies in the community working together, and (5) reasonable goals set by members of the collaborative group.

EXHIBIT 7.4
Collaborative
Arrangements
in Obesity
Prevention

Types of Collaborative Arrangements
Referral
Colocation
Purchase of services
Backbone organization
Joint advocacy for the intervention
No exchange of resources

Putting the Pieces Together

For any specific intervention aimed at obesity prevention, a variety of roles or collaborative arrangements may be carried out by partnering organizations. These arrangements include referral, colocation, purchase of services, service as a backbone organization, and joint advocacy activities (see exhibit 7.4).

The full conceptual framework conceived by Charlie and Kris is based around leveraging the opportunity provided by the joint CHNA; working through shared efforts between LHDs, local healthcare partners, and other partners, such as the school system; serving as a foundation for further collaborative relationships aimed at obesity prevention; and using concrete data to measure progress that can be shared among institutions and with members of the community. The framework is summarized in exhibit 7.5.

EXHIBIT 7.5
Framework
for Building
Effective
Cross-Sector
Collaboration

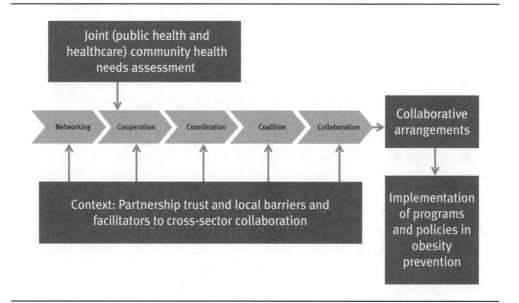

Next Steps

Charlie and Kris are excited about the possibilities of creating a community-wide effort to prevent obesity in children. They know the long-term outcomes will take time, but they also know that the initiative needs to begin immediately! They outline the next steps, with a timetable of two months:

- Develop a draft vision statement that can be used to inspire collaboration among organizations and participation among community members. The vision statement may be refined by the participating organizations once the group is formed.

- Gather descriptive statistics about the population, including demographics and as much health and behavioral health data as possible.

- If healthcare is the main focus of the intervention, gather data on the healthcare workforce, installations, and the population covered, as well as the common primary care practices in the prevention of obesity for prenatal life, children, and adults.

- If the community is also a focus of the intervention, gather data on (1) the obesity-influencing characteristics of the community, including environmental factors such as grocery stores, parks, trails, and open areas on school grounds, and (2) obesity-focused public health programs and strategies at local, regional, and state levels.

- Gather descriptive statistics about the children served by the school district, including demographics and as much health and behavioral health data as possible.

- If schools are also a focus of the intervention, gather data on the characteristics of each school in the district, including environmental factors.

- Identify a short list of key stakeholders and a longer list of additional community agencies that might become involved.

- Develop a brief description of the proposed collaborative initiative—including goals and measures of success pertaining to children and to the organizational performance—to be used to seek input and approval from the respective governing authorities.

- Convene the stakeholder organizations to refine the vision statement and gain institutional and resource support before selecting a specific intervention or digging further into operational details.

- Search for potential funding sources to cover the expenses of the planning process for the new program.

- Develop a succinct reporting format that could be shared and used by all stakeholder organizations, and that can be used by the Centennial Health Department in its application to PHAB for accreditation.

Questions

Fact and Data Analysis Questions

1. What are some sources of data on demographics, health status, and health behaviors of children and adults?
2. What characteristics of a community, healthcare, and schools might be relevant to obesity prevention measures? How, and from what sources of data, might the desired data about those characteristics be gathered?
3. What organizations might be on the list of key stakeholder organizations that Charlie and Kris created for the obesity prevention initiative? What other organizations might be on a secondary list of interested or involved organizations from the community?
4. What measures could be used over time to track changes in childhood obesity? How would these data be gathered?
5. Create Charlie and Kris's respective lists of evidence-based programs (government and private) that exist at the federal, state, local, and school district levels related to childhood nutrition, exercise, and food security.

Discussion Questions

1. If prevention is one of the ten essential functions of public health, why is a local health department unable to solve the obesity problem on its own?
2. How has accreditation by the Public Health Accreditation Board affected the activities of state and local health departments?
3. What factors have contributed to public health, personal healthcare, healthcare, and education being "separate spheres"?
4. Find two examples of community collaborative initiatives that have worked for five or more years and two that have failed. What factors lead to the success or failure of a collaborative effort? Is healthcare-related collaboration different from collaboration in other business endeavors?
5. Why would the Centers for Disease Control and Prevention sponsor research on organizational issues such as collaboration rather than on health conditions?
6. What resources will be needed to implement the three frameworks of collaboration? How will Charlie, Kris, and their respective boards know if this use of resources is beneficial to enhancing the effectiveness of the new obesity prevention initiatives?

References

American Academy of Pediatrics Council on Sports Medicine and Fitness and Council on School Health. 2006. "Active Healthy Living: Prevention of Childhood Obesity Through Increased Physical Activity." *Pediatrics* 117 (5): 1834–42.

Amherst H. Wilder Foundation. 2019. "Collaboration Factors Inventory." Accessed June 14. www.wilder.org/wilder-research/resources-and-tools#collaboration.

Boyle, M., S. Lawrence, L. Schwarte, S. Samuels, and W. J. McCarthy. 2009. "Health Care Providers' Perceived Role in Changing Environments to Promote Healthy Eating and Physical Activity: Baseline Findings from Health Care Providers Participating in the Healthy Eating, Active Communities Program." *Pediatrics* 123 (Suppl. 5): S293–S300.

Centers for Disease Control and Prevention (CDC). 2019. "CDC Community Health Improvement Navigator." Accessed February 20. wwwn.cdc.gov/chidatabase.

———. 2018. "The Public Health System & the 10 Essential Public Health Services." Reviewed June 26. www.cdc.gov/publichealthgateway/publichealthservices/essentialhealthservices.html.

Community Guide. 2019. *The Guide to Community Preventive Services.* Accessed June 14. www.thecommunityguide.org/.

Conduent Healthy Communities Institute. 2019. "Promising Practices." Accessed February 19. http://cdc.thehcn.net/.

County Health Rankings & Roadmaps. 2016. *2016 County Health Rankings Key Findings Report.* Accessed June 13. www.countyhealthrankings.org/reports/2016-county-health-rankings-key-findings-report.

Dietz, W., J. Lee, H. Wechsler, S. Malepati, and B. Sherry. 2007. "Health Plans' Role in Preventing Overweight in Children and Adolescents." *Health Affairs* 26 (2): 430–40.

Dietz, W. H., L. S. Solomon, N. Pronk, S. K. Ziegenhorn, M. Standish, M. M. Longjohn, D. D. Fukazawa, I. U. Eneli, L. Loy, N. D. Muth, E. J. Sanchez, J. Bogard, and D. W. Bradley. 2015. "An Integrated Framework for the Prevention and Treatment of Obesity and Its Related Chronic Diseases." *Health Affairs* 34 (9): 1456–63.

Frey, B., J. Lohmeier, S. Lee, and N. Tellefson. 2006. "Measuring Collaboration Among Grant Partners." *American Journal of Evaluation* 27 (3): 383–92.

Harvard T.H. Chan School of Public Health. 2019. "Obesity Prevention Source." Accessed February 19. www.hsph.harvard.edu/obesity-prevention-source/obesity-prevention/healthcare/.

Institute of Medicine (IOM). 2012. *Primary Care and Public Health: Exploring Integration to Improve Population Health.* Washington, DC: National Academies Press.

Institute of Medicine and National Research Council. 2009. *Local Government Actions to Prevent Childhood Obesity.* Washington, DC: National Academies Press.

Khan, L. K., K. Sobush, D. Keener, K. Goodman, A. Lowry, J. Kakietek, and S. Zaro. 2009. "Recommended Community Strategies and Measurements to Prevent Obesity in the United States." Centers for Disease Control and Prevention *Morbidity and Mortality Weekly Report.* Published July 24. www.cdc.gov/mmwr/preview/mmwrhtml/rr5807a1.htm.

National Association of County and City Health Officials (NACCHO). 2015. "Public Health Transformation Sentinel Network Findings from Year 1 (2014–2015)." Accessed June 13, 2019. www.naccho.org/uploads/downloadable-resources/NACCHO-Sentinel-Network-Year-1-Report_Final-2.pdf.

Obesity Society. 2010. *Position Statement: Youth Weight Bias and Discrimination in Healthcare Settings.* Silver Spring, MD: Obesity Society.

Office of the Surgeon General. 2010. *The Surgeon General's Vision for a Healthy and Fit Nation 2010.* Rockville, MD: US Department of Health and Human Services.

Rosenbaum, S. 2011. "The Patient Protection and Affordable Care Act: Implications for Public Health Policy and Practice." *Public Health Reports* 126 (1): 130–35.

Stamatakis, K. A., S. T. Leatherdale, C. M. Marx, Y. Yan, G. A. Colditz, and R. C. Brownson. 2012. "Where Is Obesity Prevention on the Map? Distribution and Predictors of Local Health Department Prevention Activities in Relation to County-Level Obesity Prevalence in the United States." *Journal of Public Health Management and Practice* 18 (5): 402–11.

White-Cooper, S., N. U. Dawkins, S. L. Kamin, and L. A. Anderson. 2009. "Community–Institutional Partnerships: Understanding Trust Among Partners." *Health Education & Behavior* 36 (2): 334–47.

Yoshida, Y., and E. J. Simoes. 2018. "Sugar-Sweetened Beverage, Obesity, and Type 2 Diabetes in Children and Adolescents: Policies, Taxation, and Programs." *Current Diabetes Reports* 18 (6): 31.

Useful Resources

- Centers for Disease Control and Prevention—Behavioral Risk Factor Surveillance System (www.cdc.gov/brfss)
- National Association of County and City Health Officials (www.naccho.org)
- Public Health Accreditation Board (www.phaboard.org)

POPULATION HEALTH

As originally articulated in 1997, *population health* refers to "the health of a population as measured by health status indicators and as influenced by social, economic, and physical environments, personal health practices, individual capacity and coping skills, human biology, early childhood development, and health services" (Government of Canada 2012). The description continues: "As an approach, population health focuses on the interrelated conditions and factors that influence the health of populations over the life course, identifies systematic variations in the patterns of occurrence, and applies the resulting knowledge to develop and implement policies and actions to improve the health and well-being of those populations" (Government of Canada 2012).

Kindig and Stoddart (2003, 380) define *population health* as "the health outcomes of a group of individuals, including the distribution of such outcomes within the group." They also note that the field of population health requires attention to multiple determinants of health outcomes and variations in observed patterns, with those findings applied for the purpose of improving the well-being of the population. This description is consistent with the concept of *population health management*, described by McAlearney (2003), which involves tracking and intervening in the health status of a specific group of people where the denominator and numerator are known. Managed care plans provide an example of organizations that have the authority, data, and incentives to engage in active management of the health of an identifiable segment of the population. Though *population health* and *population health management* have distinct meanings, the two terms are often conflated in discussions of the US system today.

Many important functions of population health have been discussed in the earlier sections of this book. Therefore, in this section, we provide a brief overview of the topic and build on the material presented already.

The Pursuit of Population Health

Critical organizational elements affect how an organization pursues population health. The most important is the way the mission, vision, values, and culture of the organization (often referred to as the "directional strategies") interface with what the organization hopes to achieve. Is population health being pursued to achieve regulatory compliance (e.g., for completion of Internal Revenue Service Form 990, Schedule H), to attain accreditation (e.g., to gain National Cancer Institute designation), or to improve financial or quality metrics as advanced by value-based quality payment adjustments to providers? Or is the pursuit simply a reflection of the organization's mission and fundamental culture (e.g., the Catholic Health Association's commitment to community benefit)? In many instances, population health efforts are driven by an amalgamation of multiple factors.

The organization's directional strategies and what the organization hopes to achieve influence the definition of the population and the prism through which the population is viewed. A population can be defined by age, income, geography, community, employer, insurance coverage, health status (mental or physical), or some combination of factors (Nash et al. 2015; Riegelman 2019). For example, a population might consist of diabetic patients in a particular county who are Medicaid eligible. Multiple criteria are commonly employed as a pragmatic means of focusing programmatic efforts.

As the population is defined, assets and community resources related to the defined population must be ascertained. The assets, organizations, and people identified will serve as partners and collaborators, as well as stakeholders, to leverage in improving the health and well-being of the population.

After the target population has been defined and relevant assets of the community have been determined, the process of influencing the health of the population enters into the analytical phase. At this point, patterns, anomalies, and outliers are identified. Biostatistical, health informatic, and epidemiological skills are helpful when teasing out opportunities to improve (Caron 2017). Data sets must be examined, or created, that extend beyond those traditionally used by hospitals and physicians, to incorporate information available through public health programs, environmental health, acute care, long-term care, and community-based systems. A person's electronic health record already includes zip code, demographic and lifestyle data, as well as clinical care and health status data.

As trends and opportunities emerge, reexamination of the mission and vision of the organization can help guide prioritization of possible interventions. In some instances, the population health issues identified in the analysis may be merely tangential to the purpose and mission of the organization, may move the organization away from its core business, or may require essential competencies that the organization itself does not possess. As a result, the proposed population health initiative may require adjustment before moving on to the next steps. The steps to this point are nonlinear and may undergo multiple iterations.

Several frameworks have been advanced to provide insight into how institutional and community mechanisms can be leveraged to influence change. Examples include the social determinants of health framework, the Health Belief Model, Andersen's Healthcare Utilization Model, and the Ecological Model of Health. What these models have in common is a movement beyond medical care and away from the Epidemiological

Triangle to include social and community factors that influence health, as well as the responsible agents, psychological factors, policies, financial factors, and existing individual-level incentives.

The models and analytics should help identify a number of factors (both root cause and contributing) driving the observed patterns or anomalies of health status and healthcare service use. Once it has identified the causes and applied the theories of change, the organization can develop an intervention and put a health improvement plan in place. To be effective, components of the plan should address the relevant psychological, social cohesion, socioeconomic, physical environment, economic, genetic, and disparity factors, in addition to elements more closely related to medical care.

Programs that have documented evidence of success with the chosen target audience are generally preferable to interventions that lack such evidence—unless the organization is engaged in research or seeks to pilot and evaluate innovations. The development of a detailed implementation plan and a sustainable management plan will drive partnerships, engage multiple stakeholders, and create a burning platform that encourages long-term participation.

Population health management interventions and improvement plans are typically oriented toward lifestyle management, demand management, disease management, catastrophic care, or disability (McAlearney 2003). Lifestyle management is concerned with individual risk reduction and health promotion via education, motivation, training, or marketing (Elder, Geller, and Mayer 1993). Demand management initiatives use decision support services—with regard to provider selection or end-of-life care, for instance—to influence the way individuals make healthcare decisions (Vickery 1996). Disease management focuses on coordination of care across the healthcare spectrum, though it also includes aspects of both lifestyle management and demand management (McAlearney 2003). Catastrophic care can be considered a subset of disease management, focused specifically on areas where the costs, acuity, and complexity of cases are high. Dedicated infrastructure, training, and resources are often associated with catastrophic care management. Finally, disability management is concerned with the reduction of costs associated with and the incidence of disability in a given population. Initiatives of all these types involve capturing data about a population both before and after an intervention, as well as having a benchmark or standard as a desired outcome.

New-era population health programs may be aimed at changing factors in the environment, society, culture, or community for which precise metrics about individual participants are not known or available. These more global efforts leapfrog the collection of data pertaining to the short-term impact on individuals and take a longer view of changes that can be made to population groups. The logic model is less precise, but the focus on long-term outcomes is consistent with recognition of the impact of social determinants of health, as measured at the community level, on the health of an individual.

Regardless of the approach pursued, population health management necessitates moving beyond the focus on continuous quality improvement in the delivery of episodic or acute care provided by doctors or hospitals; it requires the involvement of employers, schools, social services, government, and public health organizations that have a stake in improving the health of the population (Kindig 1998). Improvement plans should be clearly defined, and they should incorporate the managerial science surrounding effectiveness and sustainability. Measures of quality extend beyond clinical care to include quality of the environment (e.g., air quality, food security, walkability), attitudes of society (e.g., lifestyle factors, life satisfaction scores), and other more global concepts.

Finally, evaluation of programs and attribution of improvements to particular initiatives are challenging but important functions for an organization or individual pursuing population health. The analytical stage should be revisited to assemble feedback about the effectiveness of the plan, partners, and initiatives. The findings allow for promotion of initiatives that work, initiatives that make a difference on the desired metrics, and initiatives that warrant the allocation of institutional resources; they also allow for the discontinuation of initiatives that provide more limited benefit. Evaluation of partnership efficacy is also critical, as advocated by the collective impact movement.

Throughout the iterative and nonlinear process of managing population health (summarized in exhibit 1), individuals and organizations must rely on foundational competencies related to leadership, management, directional strategies, analytics, and communication. They also must engage in advocacy at the local, state, and federal levels to support the underlying goals of the organization and to help improve the community's health status and healthcare system.

The Cases

As in the earlier sections of this book, the cases in this section present health challenges that extend beyond a single organization. Large-scale population health efforts are highly complex, and they require multi-institutional, multidimensional approaches with the resources necessary to sustain them over time.

In case 8, an acute care center and a community service organization explore the development of a model—perhaps an accountable care organization—to provide infrastructure, staff, and financing to assist people with spinal cord injuries.

Case 9 focuses on efforts by the Veterans Health Administration (VHA) to improve its approach to caring for veterans, particularly as the veteran population ages. The case considers ways in which the VHA can work with organizations in the community to meet the needs of aging seniors in a cost-effective, high-quality manner.

Case 10 looks at the broad community-oriented programs sponsored by Rush Medical Center in Chicago, where myriad challenges related to social determinants of health affect local population subgroups.

Finally, case 11 highlights a program in Phoenix, Arizona, that seeks to address the tragedy of homelessness for local residents while also improving the use of the health system's scarce resources.

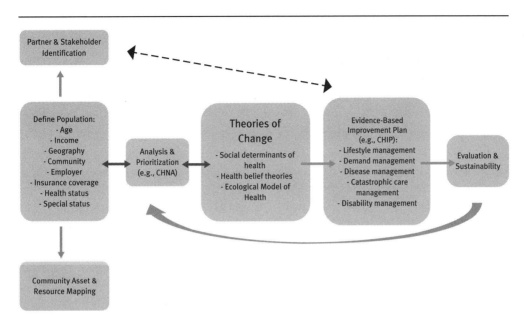

EXHIBIT 1
The Process
of Managing
Population
Health

References

Caron, R. M. 2017. *Population Health: Principles and Applications for Management.* Chicago: Health Administration Press.

Elder, J. P., E. S. Geller, and J. A. Mayer. 1993. *Motivating Health Behavior.* Clifton Park, NY: Delmar Cengage Learning.

Government of Canada. 2012. "What Is the Population Health Approach?" Modified February 7. www.canada.ca/en/public-health/services/health-promotion/population-health/population-health-approach.html.

Kindig, D. A. 1998. "Purchasing Population Health: Aligning Financial Incentives to Improve Health Outcomes." *Health Services Research* 33 (2 pt. 1): 223–42.

Kindig, D., and G. Stoddart. 2003. "What Is Population Health?" *American Journal of Public Health* 93 (3): 380–83.

McAlearney, A. S. 2003. *Population Health Management: Strategies to Improve Outcomes.* Chicago: Health Administration Press.

Nash, D. B., R. J. Fabius, A. Skoufalos, J. L. Clark, and M. R. Horowitz. 2015. *Population Health: Creating a Culture of Wellness,* 2nd ed. Burlington, MA: Jones & Bartlett Learning.

Riegelman, R. 2019. *Population Health: A Primer.* Burlington, MA: Jones & Bartlett Learning.

Vickery, D. M. 1996. "Demand Management. Toward Appropriate Use of Medical Care." *Healthcare Forum Journal* 39 (1): 14–19.

COORDINATING CARE FOR SPECIAL POPULATIONS: FACILITATING CARE COORDINATION AND CARE TRANSITION FOR PEOPLE WITH MOBILITY LIMITATIONS

Reena Joseph, Tapan Mehta, James H. Rimmer, Charles L. Angel Jr., Jamie Wade, and Allyson Hall

Case at a Glance

Overarching theme

This case focuses on how to develop operational coordination among separate institutions to create a system that is effective and efficient in meeting the multifaceted needs of people with complex chronic conditions, within the constraints of the US health insurance model.

Learning objectives

- Define *disability*.
- Characterize the subgroups of people with disabilities.
- Explain the rehabilitation components of the US health system.
- Compare public and private insurance programs with regard to coverage for rehabilitation services.
- Explain the rationale for offering select populations with disabilities a comprehensive continuum of care, including social and mental health as well as standard health services.
- Critique the criteria used to determine eligibility for Supplemental Security Income and disability insurance.
- Contrast the methods for linking clinical case management across discrete health service provider organizations.
- Articulate the issues involved in sharing clinical and administrative information across health service provider organizations.
- Analyze the foundations necessary to build an accountable care organization, or comparable program, that integrates service and financing.

Key terms	• Accountable care organization (ACO) • Americans with Disabilities Act • Case management • Disability • Medicaid • Medicare • Rehabilitation • Rehabilitation hospital • Social Security Administration • Spinal cord injury (SCI) • Supplemental insurance
Management competencies	Health services and systems, organizational behavior, financial management
Population/ subgroup	People who have spinal cord injuries and others needing rehabilitation
Health issue or condition	Spinal cord injuries

Management Challenge

Treatment for patients with traumatic spinal cord injuries (SCIs) is highly complex and extremely expensive, and it requires coordination among various providers across the care continuum. Patients with SCIs face mobility limitations and long-term disability, are increasingly likely to develop secondary health complications, and have more frequent hospital emergency department (ED) visits and unplanned hospital readmissions. The movement of such patients across the rehabilitation continuum is further complicated by differences in the number of allowable rehabilitation visits under various insurance plans.

The Spencer Center is a rehabilitation unit within the Regional Academic Health System (RAHS), and the Community Rehab Foundation (CRF) is a not-for-profit organization focused on improving the lives of people with physical disabilities. Together, the organizations are interested in developing a care coordination and care transition program that will enable patients with traumatic SCIs to transition seamlessly from the acute care center back into the community, enhancing quality of care and reducing the incidence of hospital readmission. An additional step might be to create an accountable care organization (ACO) under the Center for Medicare & Medicaid Services (CMS) Center for Innovation. An ACO model could provide a financial package to cover the costs of coordinated, comprehensive care. Measures of quality as well as financial performance are essential to an ACO's success.

The CEOs of the RAHS Spencer Center and CRF have created a task force to start the process of collaboration and to explore the possibility of forming an ACO.

Background

Spinal Cord Injury

Spinal cord injury refers to any damage to the spinal cord or nerves within the spinal canal resulting in temporary or permanent loss of movement and/or feeling. SCIs may be acute, resulting from a traumatic event, or they may be the result of chronic degenerative disease.

The National Spinal Cord Injury Statistical Center (NSCISC 2019) estimates the prevalence of SCIs in the United States to be approximately 291,000 individuals, with 17,000 new cases each year. The most common causes of SCIs are motor vehicle accidents, accidental falls, sport-related injuries, and violent acts. The average age at injury is 43 years. Falls are the most common cause of traumatic SCIs among individuals aged 65 years or older. Less than 1 percent of SCI cases experience complete neurological recovery by the time of hospital discharge—which underscores the importance of proper rehabilitation.

About 30 percent of individuals with SCIs are rehospitalized one or more times during any given year following injury, with nearly 55 percent being rehospitalized during the first year (Cardenas et al. 2004; Richards et al. 2017). The average length of stay is 22 days; the stay is longer for people using a wheelchair than for those who are able to walk. The most common causes of readmissions for people with SCIs are skin diseases (e.g., pressure ulcers) and infections of the genitourinary system. Other causes of SCI-related readmissions and secondary health complications are diseases of the respiratory, digestive, musculoskeletal, and circulatory systems.

Common Examples of Spinal Cord Injuries

- Marco was driving home from a bar downtown. Having consumed a significant amount of alcohol, he lost focus and began drifting out of his lane. Upon realizing he was on the shoulder of the road, Marco overcorrected and collided with Craig, a motorcyclist. Craig broke his neck in the accident and lost function of all four limbs. Auto accidents are the leading cause of SCIs each year (NSCISC 2019).
- A 67-year-old woman named Rose slipped and fell at her neighbor's house while coming down the stairs. The stairs were wet from the rain and did not have a handrail. Slip-and-fall accidents account for a large portion of SCIs each year (NSCISC 2019). Injury is most common in falls after the age of 65.
- Carly was at her local swimming pool during the summer. Despite warning signs about shallow water, Carly dove in headfirst. She hit the bottom of the pool and suffered an SCI, becoming paraplegic. Sports accidents are another common cause of SCIs (NSCISC 2019).

In 2018, the average annual expenses (including healthcare costs and living expenses) associated with SCIs ranged from nearly $370,000 to $1,130,000 in the first year, depending on type of injury, extent of neurological impairment, and education (NSCISC 2019). In the same year, the indirect costs in terms of lost wages, benefits, and productivity averaged about $76,000 per patient. Healthcare providers are interested in changing the payment model used for SCIs. Value-based models tend to penalize hospitals and physicians if a patient is readmitted frequently or too soon after discharge. A new payment model, ideally, would balance the clinical needs of people with SCIs with adequate compensation for those who provide care for them.

People with permanent SCIs may qualify as "permanently disabled" according to the Social Security Administration and become eligible for Medicare health insurance and Supplemental Security Income. CMS therefore has a financial interest in creating ACOs to provide effective, efficient care for people with disabilities.

Prominent Individuals with Spinal Cord Injuries

- "Superman" actor Christopher Reeve suffered an SCI in 1995 when he was thrown off a horse during an equestrian competition. He broke his neck in the fall and became quadriplegic. He later became an advocate for people with SCIs and a champion for research on SCI recovery.
- Martial artist, actor, and stuntman Jackie Chan has suffered numerous injuries throughout his career. During the filming of his 1985 movie *Police Story,* a fall from a pole left him with spinal damage and a pelvis dislocation, almost causing partial paralysis. Ultimately, he recovered and faced no permanent damage.
- Canadian athlete Rick Hansen was thrown from the back of a pick-up truck when he was 15 years old, suffering an SCI and becoming paraplegic. In 1985, he embarked on his Man in Motion World Tour, traveling through more than 30 countries in his wheelchair. A three-time Paralympic Games gold medalist, he was inducted into Canada's Sports Hall of Fame in 2006.
- Roy Campanella, a star for the Brooklyn Dodgers in the 1940s and 1950s, is widely considered one of the best catchers in the history of baseball. In 1958, he was in a serious car accident, fracturing several vertebrae and compressing his spinal cord. Initially paralyzed from the shoulders down, he was able to regain use of his arms and hands through therapy. Campanella was inducted into the Baseball Hall of Fame in 1969.
- Charles Krauthammer was a first-year medical student at Harvard Medical School when he experienced an SCI while diving into a swimming pool. He severed his spinal cord at the C5 vertebrae and became paralyzed from the waist down. Krauthammer completed medical school and became a psychiatrist, husband, and father—and later a news analyst, political commentator, and author. He won a Pulitzer Prize for Commentary in 1987.

The Regional Academic Health System

The Regional Academic Health System is a large academic health center in the Mid-western United States that has been included in *U.S. News and World Report*'s rankings of best hospitals, the list of the 100 best hospitals in America, and the list of the "most wired" hospitals. Within RAHS is a dedicated rehabilitation facility called the Spencer Center. A licensed specialty rehabilitation hospital, the Spencer Center is recognized as one of the foremost providers of comprehensive physical medicine and rehabilitation in the Midwest. The 45-bed center has treated more than 400,000 patients since opening in the late 1960s. Patients come from throughout the Midwest and the South; a small number come from other countries.

The Spencer Center is a hub for the Spinal Cord Injury Model System, a nationally recognized approach for providing multidisciplinary rehabilitation care, from emergency services through rehabilitation and reentry into full community life. The Model System was sponsored by the National Institute on Disability, Independent Living, and Rehabilitation Research (NIDILRR), which supports innovative research in the delivery, demonstration, and evaluation of medical, rehabilitation, vocational, and other services to meet the needs of individuals with SCIs (Administration for Community Living 2019; Model Systems Knowledge Translation Center 2019).

Services offered at the Spencer Center include the following:

- Physical therapy
- Occupational therapy
- Speech therapy
- Balance and vestibular training
- Prostheses fitting and maintenance
- Locomotor training
- Rehabilitation pool and water-based exercises
- Driver rehabilitation

The Spencer Center and RAHS work synergistically to care for patients in the immediate period following an SCI event. Services are typically covered by insurance; most are provided on a short-term basis. Once patients advance to a stable clinical condition or use up the amount of rehabilitation services covered by their insurance, they are responsible for paying for services out-of-pocket—even if the SCI causes them to lose their job (and job-related health insurance).

New models of care for people with SCIs are being extensively researched nation-wide. One such model involves an ACO structure, developed under the auspices of the CMS Center for Innovation. In an ACO, doctors and other providers come together to coordinate care and share financial risk for a defined population. Measures of patient medical expense and quality, in addition to shared structural risk between entities, determine whether the ACO makes or loses money. Shared-risk arrangements with CMS indicate the level of risk the ACO agrees to assume. (Further information about current risk models is available through the CMS website at www.cms.gov.)

Community Rehab Foundation

The Community Rehab Foundation is a not-for-profit organization dedicated to improving the lives of individuals with physical disabilities. It provides community-based sport, fitness, and therapeutic recreation programs, as well as advocacy, policy, and research activities. Designated by the official US Olympic Committee as an Olympic and Paralympic Training Site, CRF serves more than 4,000 unique individuals every year. Payment for services comes from a variety of sources, including self-pay, third-party commercial insurance, select government programs, grants from foundations, donations, and any other source that CRF can tap. Like the Spencer Center, CRF is heavily involved in research for SCI models of care. It would likely benefit from working with the center to create an ACO.

Collaboration

At present, no formal agreement exists between Spencer Center and CRF for the transfer of patients. Patients frequently go to CRF to meet their ongoing rehabilitation needs after their initial rehabilitation at Spencer Center is complete, and clients of CRF often go to RAHS if they experience acute medical problems. If a patient goes to the Spencer Center, the staff there are likely to know the staff at CRF. However, if a patient simply appears in the RAHS ED in the middle of the night, the staff on duty might not be aware of CRF and the additional resources it may be providing to the patient. Both the Spencer Center and CRF have their own clinical information systems (both use independently tailored versions of EPIC), financial contracts with third-party payers, and internal methods for care coordination.

Care coordination across service providers is challenging and complex. To gain a better understanding of the issue, CRF tasked two interns with conducting a detailed review of best practices in care coordination and care transition programs for patients with traumatic SCIs. The review indicated that current programs included a number of discrete components, such as longer rehabilitation, vocational training, and the use of community resources, but that no comprehensive strategy had been developed for patient care transition between a major health system and a dedicated community-based organization.

One major barrier to coordination across SCI-related service providers is that insurance coverage for patients with SCIs varies greatly from one payer to another. For instance, Medicaid coverage for SCIs varies from state to state, with some states providing extensive coverage (including attendant care, community support coordination, occupational therapy, physical therapy, and residential rehabilitation) and other states covering only a more restrictive list of services. Significant variation also exists in the rehabilitation benefits provided by private insurance plans, such as allowed days of coverage for inpatient and outpatient rehabilitation, assignment of a designated case manager, and annual or lifetime limits on number of days of rehabilitation.

Formal collaboration between the RAHS Spencer Center and CRF would likely help both organizations, as well as their clients with SCIs. Managing people with SCIs as a population might allow for bundling services and spreading risk across everyone in the population, rather than paying for each individual client with unique service use. However, determining how to structure the collaboration to mutually benefit the two organizations and determining what processes will be used, by whom, and when require considerable planning and commitment of resources from the organizations' governing boards.

Patient Perspective Excerpts

In addition to physical problems, people with spinal cord injuries experience an array of social, financial, and emotional challenges. Upon experiencing an SCI, highly independent people with good jobs and solid incomes can suddenly become impoverished, and family members may suddenly find themselves as caregivers. Addressing such a broad range of problems can be overwhelming, and patients and their families often turn to the healthcare system for physical, emotional, or functional support.

Executives of the Spencer Center and CRF conducted a survey of patients and families to generate useful information with which to establish a rationale and priorities for creating a comprehensive and unified service path. Asked about their recent SCIs, clients made the following comments:

- Client 1: "I had the family support I needed, but I did not have the financial support to get the most out of the state and federally funded programs. I did not have any insurance. I got hit by a drunk driver and there was a lawsuit, but we didn't get any financial compensation. There was an insurance settlement that paid the hospital bills, but other than that, I only had the state-funded rehab program."
- Client 2: "I was assigned a counselor whom I could call, but I can't remember anyone coming to my house. I would have expected at least that level of involvement. . . . Plus, if there are programs available to help, I would hope that someone would make sure you have access to them so that you can take care of yourself."
- Client 3: "I had a great experience at the rehab center. My physical therapist came back home with me to speak to the school, my class, and my work, and gave a general lecture about spinal cord injury and disability. The people in our community really came in and helped, like building a ramp into the house."

(continued)

- Caregiver 1: "Orchestrating all the services that my husband needed when he was discharged from the Spencer Center with an SCI was a full-time job. I had to quit my real job to take care of him—which then caused additional financial strain on our family. CRF was very helpful in providing information about available services, providing some services directly, and making contact with other services. Equally important, CRF encouraged my husband, my family, and me to keep a positive attitude during this difficult time."
- Caregiver 2: "Our family went from healthy, happy, solid income to permanent disability, no income, fear, and depression. I had never heard of 'ADLs' or 'IADLs.' The road to independent functioning is hardly clear and very lonely. When there is a problem, I don't know where to turn, so we go to the emergency department at the hospital and eventually make our way back to the Spencer Center."
- Client 4: "The Spencer Center used to have a recreational therapist who would take patients out into the public, to movies or bowling or activities outside of the hospital. But they did away with that program when I got there. . . . That is one thing I would suggest—that they let patients go out of the hospital and experience things outside of the four walls. I think rehab places need to have that."
- Client 5: "When I went to rehab, they had a very high census, and the therapists were not able to spend too long with one patient. So, I had a lot of downtime. When I went there as an inpatient, I had a hard time getting in. They did not even have a room for me. I guess a lot of people need rehabilitation, and there is not enough capacity to take care of everyone when they need help."

Task Force Objectives

The CEOs of the Spencer Center and CRF outline the following priorities for the task force:

- Develop a conceptual framework that depicts movement of the SCI patient across the care continuum, from injury to reintegration back into the community.
- Propose organizational processes and procedures that both the Spencer Center and CRF can employ to achieve seamless transition of SCI patients back into the community.
- Identify key stakeholders in this process, along with the role(s) that each stakeholder would play.

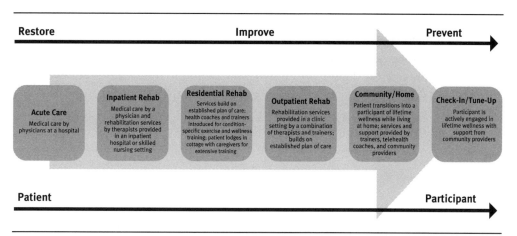

EXHIBIT 8.1
Vision for
the Spinal
Cord Injury
Continuum of
Care

- Build a business case for the collaboration, such that the services from both organizations can be billed to the patient's insurer and the RAHS Spencer Center can participate in value-based payment systems appropriate for the management of populations needing rehabilitation.

The CEOs would like this work to be completed within three months—six at the most—and they each are considering the "next steps" to get this process underway. First, they need to create the vision that will lead to the "elevator speech" to sell their organizations' governing bodies on the merits of the project. To provide a starting point, CRF has offered a graphic display of its vision of a continuum of care for people needing rehabilitation (see exhibit 8.1).

Questions

Fact and Data Analysis Questions

1. What conditions other than spinal cord injuries cause people to use rehabilitation services?
2. How many dollars are spent each year on physical therapy, occupational therapy, and speech therapy? What proportion of total annual healthcare expenditures are spent on rehabilitation?
3. What is the total number of rehabilitation hospitals in the United States? Where else are rehabilitation services provided?
4. What rehabilitation services are covered, and within what limits, by Medicare? By Medicaid?
5. What are the National Institutes of Health (NIH)? How are they structured? Where does rehabilitation fit into the NIH?

6. What is the Americans with Disabilities Act? What are the implications of the law for a person with an SCI?

7. How does one qualify for Supplemental Security Income? Describe the criteria and the process.

8. How, if at all, would an ACO model help people with SCIs?

9. What measures of quality of care, as used by CMS, apply to the care of people with SCIs?

10. What factors would mitigate financial risk for the sponsoring organizations in an ACO for people with SCIs?

Discussion Questions

1. What challenges do clients with rehabilitation needs face in accessing the full set of services that would benefit them?

2. What do the comments from patients and caregivers (see text box) reveal about the rehabilitation system in general?

3. What are some problems that may result when payers only cover rehabilitation services that they deem "medically necessary"? What are the long-term implications for patients with physical disabilities?

4. Define *case management*. What types of healthcare professionals provide it? How is it paid for? How has case management evolved over the past 50 years?

5. What is the role of the US federal government in advancing new models of care? Consider programs of the National Institutes of Health, the Centers for Disease Control and Prevention, the Agency for Healthcare Research and Quality, and CMS, among others. How are prototype models expanded beyond pilot projects?

6. As Medicare and private insurers move to bundled payment models, what bundles include rehabilitation services?

7. Compare the way the Spencer Center and CRF interact now with the way they would interact if a more formal arrangement for collaboration were in place. What basic parameters would be essential to a formal collaboration?

8. Is an ACO framework consistent with the SCI vision of a continuum of care? How could an ACO facilitate or impede implementation of the vision?

9. If the Spencer Center and CRF want to determine the full cost of caring for a person with an SCI, what data should the participating entities share? What information from additional organizations would be needed to get a complete picture of all expenses? What are the information system implications or requirements? What confidentiality requirements address the sharing of patient data across organizations?

10. What items on the task force's list need to be completed before planning for a joint ACO can begin?

References

Administration for Community Living (ACL). 2019. "About the National Institute on Disability, Independent Living, and Rehabilitation Research (NIDILRR)." Modified April 26. https://acl.gov/about-acl/about-national-institute-disability-independent-living-and-rehabilitation-research.

Cardenas, D. D., J. M. Hoffman, S. Kirshblum, and W. McKinley. 2004. "Etiology and Incidence of Rehospitalization After Traumatic Spinal Cord Injury: A Multicenter Analysis." *Archives of Physical Medicine and Rehabilitation* 85 (11): 1757–63.

Model Systems Knowledge Translation Center. 2019. "Directory of Model Systems." Accessed June 17. https://msktc.org/sci/model-system-centers.

National Spinal Cord Injury Statistical Center (NSCISC). 2019. "Spinal Cord Injury (SCI) Facts and Figures at a Glance." Accessed June 17. www.nscisc.uab.edu/Public/Facts%20and%20Figures%202019%20-%20Final.pdf.

Richards, C., N. MacKenzie, S. Roberts, and R. Escorpizo. 2017. "People with Spinal Cord Injury in the United States." *American Journal of Physical Medicine & Rehabilitation* 96 (2): S124–26.

Useful Resources

- Administration for Community Living—National Institute on Disability, Independent Living, and Rehabilitation Research (https://acl.gov/about-acl/about-national-institute-disability-independent-living-and-rehabilitation-research)

- American Congress of Rehabilitation Medicine—Spinal Cord Injury (https://acrm.org/acrm-communities/spinal-cord-injury/)

- American Spinal Injury Association (https://asia-spinalinjury.org)

- Centers for Disease Control and Prevention—Disability and Health (www.cdc.gov/ncbddd/disabilityandhealth/index.html)

- National Center on Health, Physical Activity, and Disability (www.nchpad.org)

- National Institute of Neurological Disorders and Stroke—Spinal Cord Injury Information Page (www.ninds.nih.gov/Disorders/All-Disorders/Spinal-Cord-Injury-Information-Page)

- National Spinal Cord Injury Statistical Center (www.nscisc.uab.edu)

SERVING SENIOR VETERANS: MANAGING COST AND QUALITY FOR HIGH-RISK AGED VETERAN POPULATIONS

Orna Intrator, Bruce Kinosian, Jim Rudolph, Ranak Trivedi, Ciaran Phibbs, and Marianne Shaughnessy

Note: The statistics in this case are intended for pedagogical purposes; some have been fabricated, and others are approximations based on past US Department of Veterans Affairs data.

Case at a Glance

Overarching theme	This case focuses on managing the health of a high-risk target population among veterans receiving care from the Veterans Health Administration, with the aim of providing high-quality care to the maximum number of veterans while minimizing costs.
Learning objectives	• Describe the organization, financing, and service array of the Veterans Health Administration. • Articulate the management issues related to meeting the needs of the aged veteran population. • Apply strategies and tools to identify high-risk populations. • Use data, assessment tools, and information systems to manage high-risk population groups. • Apply national benchmarks and models to local settings.
Key terms	• Activities of daily living (ADLs) • Frailty index • Geriatrics • Geriatrics and Extended Care (GEC) • Instrumental activities of daily living (IADLs) • Veteran • Veterans Health Administration (VHA)
Management competencies	Management of high-risk populations, quality control for care

Population/ subgroup	Veterans, senior veterans, rural populations
Health issue or condition	Chronic conditions and functional limitations

Management Challenge

Jose Lopez is the new administrator of a Veterans Health Administration (VHA) clinic in the southwestern United States. His clinic serves a population of about 300,000 across a sparsely populated desert area spanning more than 500 square miles. Meeting seniors' needs in such a setting is particularly challenging. Many seniors in the area have chronic conditions that require ongoing attention, yet they live alone, at a great distance from the clinic. Some of the veterans have to drive for three hours to see their provider.

Having come from a large VHA Medical Center in an urban area on the East Coast, Jose is aware of the various care delivery models VHA has tested in its efforts to balance optimum quality of care with affordable costs for both veterans and VHA. Jose is also familiar with the provisions of the Maintaining Internal Systems and Strengthening Integrated Outside Networks (MISSION) Act of 2018, which aims to improve

Personal Perspective

Evan is a veteran of the Vietnam War. Newly retired after 40 years of running his own business in Chicago, he has recently moved to the Southwest. Because of his arthritis, Evan had been having difficulties shoveling snow in the winter, maintaining his yard in the summer, and climbing on his roof to clean the gutters in the fall. In short, he and his wife were ready for a change. They hoped that the Southwest would provide a simpler and less expensive lifestyle, especially if they moved to one of the new communities being developed in a rural area. Since moving to the Southwest, Evan has not had any health problems, so he does not yet have a primary care physician.

About a month after getting settled, Evan seems to be tired all the time and occasionally becomes short of breath. His wife is concerned about his health, and she convinces him to see a doctor. Evan had private health insurance when he lived in Chicago, but now that he is no longer employed, he has determined that VHA will be his place for care. Evan's wife insists that they go to the Southwest Clinic, about 90 miles from their home. They head out the next morning at 8 a.m., assuming they will be seen and cared for.

veterans' access to community care (US Department of Veterans Affairs 2019c). Under the new access standards, veterans may be eligible for community care if they are a 30-minute drive from VHA outpatient services or a one-hour drive from a VHA specialty care site. Eligible veterans have the choice of using VHA services or non-VHA providers who are in the network.

Jose's challenge is to determine which, if any, care models for senior veterans will be most effective for his new clinic and the people it serves. His hope is for the clinic to be the service provider of choice among the area's veterans.

Background

The Veterans Health Administration, a component of the US Department of Veterans Affairs (VA), is the largest health system in the United States. It provides a wide range of medical, surgical, and specialty services through a system of 1,250 healthcare facilities, including 172 VA Medical Centers and 1,069 outpatient care sites (VA 2018b). Its Community-Based Outpatient Clinics (CBOCs) help make common outpatient services more easily accessible to people in rural locations. VHA serves about 9 million enrolled veterans each year (VA 2019e).

Funding for VHA is allocated annually by Congress. Despite the nation's commitment to caring for its veterans, all administrators within VHA understand that funds are tight and that care must be provided in an efficient and cost-effective manner. Population-based approaches offer the potential to maximize both quality of services and the number of veterans served, while remaining within the allowable budget.

The Aging Population

Senior veterans, defined as those aged 65 or older, make up an increasing proportion of VHA clients. Given that older adults tend to be heavy users of healthcare services, this aging of the veteran population results in higher costs. A key aspect of this trend is the wave of aging Vietnam-era veterans with complex medical, cognitive, psychosocial, and socioeconomic issues that strongly influence their healthcare needs (Clarke, Gregory, and Salomon 2015).

More than 3 million veterans enrolled in VA are age 65 or older and receive some care from VHA. Studies suggest that more than 80 percent of enrolled veterans will likely need some type of assistance with activities of daily living, and more than 55 percent of enrolled aged veterans may qualify for nursing home care (Kinosian, Stallard, and Wieland 2007). The number of veterans 65 or older is projected to rise to more than 4.5 million by 2024, and the number of veterans eligible for nursing home care to be paid by VHA will double to over 1 million (VetPop16 2017). Next to inpatient hospital care, nursing home care is the single most expensive level of care offered by VHA. Population trends and projections related to senior veterans, and older US adults in general, are shown in exhibit 9.1.

EXHIBIT 9.1
Senior
Population
Trends

Projected Population Figures (in millions)				
	2016	2020	2030	2040
Veterans—all	19.6	18.1	14.9	12.5
Veterans—age 65+	9.2	8.6	7.1	5.4
Veterans—age 85+	1.7	1.5	1.4	1.4
US—all	323.1	332.6	354.8	373.1
US—age 65+	49.2	56.1	73.1	80.8
US—age 85+	6.4	6.7	9.1	14.4

Note: Some figures have been rounded.
Source: Data from VA (2019d); Vespa, Armstrong, and Medina (2018).

VHA must serve a growing number of older veterans with increasingly severe healthcare needs, and it must do so while maintaining a balanced budget. This challenge is not unlike the difficulties faced by Medicare and many states' Medicaid programs.

Geriatrics and Extended Care

People receiving Geriatrics and Extended Care (GEC) services through VHA account for 7 percent of the veterans served and 32 percent of the total VHA budget.

The main pillars of GEC policy for veterans are access, balance, and care coordination—collectively, "the ABCs of GEC":

- *Access*—Optimizing the health, independence, and well-being of veterans by ensuring access to geriatrics, palliative care, and long-term services and supports (LTSS) in institutions, homes, and community-based settings (VA 2019a)
- *Balance*—Honoring veterans' preferences by increasing the delivery of LTSS in home and community-based settings (VA 2019a); in many cases, community-based care has been associated with reductions in preventable hospital and nursing home stays and emergency department visits, thereby reducing costs to VA (Eiken et al. 2017; Blackburn et al. 2016; Segelman et al. 2017)
- *Care coordination*—Supporting optimal care coordination and management to improve quality of care and to enhance veterans' experience as they face the challenges of aging, disability, or serious illness; coordination is especially crucial when home care is needed or during transitions between care settings (VA 2019a)

VHA has conceptualized care for seniors using the GEC continuum shown in exhibit 9.2. Care for older patients begins in ambulatory settings (on the left side of the exhibit), where evaluation and management of geriatric syndromes are performed. Such settings also offer consultation regarding palliative care. VHA has adopted a patient-centered medical home model for primary care based around units known

EXHIBIT 9.2

Continuum of Care

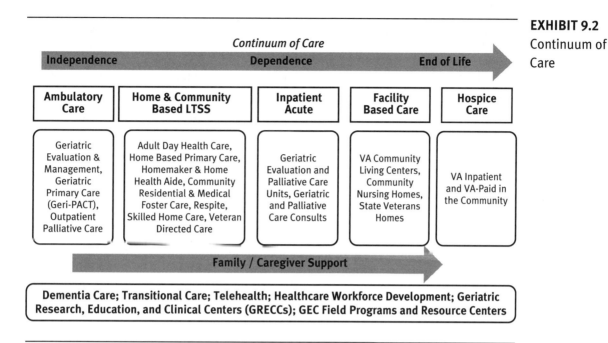

Source: Adapted from the US Department of Veterans Affairs.

as Patient Aligned Care Teams (PACTs). One type of PACT is the geriatric-focused PACT, or GeriPACT (VA 2016).

When patients are unable to perform some activities of daily living (ADLs) or instrumental activities of daily living (IADLs), or when they have challenges related to dementia, they shift to the next section of the continuum, which deals with home- and community-based LTSS. Offerings in this category may include activities through the Adult Day Health Care program, care from a Homemaker or Home Health Aide, or Respite Care service to help relieve family caregivers (VA 2018a). More extensive services include VA's Home Based Primary Care (HBPC) and Residential and Medical Foster Care.

If a patient's condition worsens and inpatient care becomes necessary, specialists in geriatric medicine can provide consultation on regular inpatient care and help address geriatric syndromes that surround acute care, such as delirium. If a patient's conditions can no longer be managed at home, the patient can receive facility-based care in nursing homes owned by VA, in state veterans homes, or through contracts with community nursing homes.

When a patient approaches the end of life, VA provides assistance in coordinating hospice care in the community. It also provides hospice care in inpatient settings, including its nursing homes. The VA Central Office (VACO) of GEC develops and manages programs that support the transition of veterans across institutional and noninstitutional settings.

VA has been an innovator of several home-based programs. The HBPC program, which was initiated in the 1970s, provides interdisciplinary team care to veterans at home (Beales and Edes 2009). In recent years, as the focus on population health has grown, a number of health systems have followed in VA's footsteps with their own models of HBPC (Reckrey et al. 2015; Leff et al. 2015; DeCherrie, Soriano, and Hayashi 2012). Another innovative VA program is the Medical Foster Home (MFH) program, in which care providers (often families) in the community take in up to three veterans and provide them with daily care under the guidance and coordination of VA's HBPC (Levy et al. 2016; Levy and Whitfield 2016). Yet another example is Veteran-Directed Care (VDC), which allows veterans to hire family and friends to care for them so they can remain at home—an option Medicare does not offer (Garrido et al. 2017; Thomas and Allen 2016).

VHA has analyzed the costs of caring for aging veterans, taking into account the various settings, and it has found that the per-person costs for people in institutional settings are significantly higher than the costs for people who receive care while residing at home. In 2017, the cost for institutional care was ten times greater than the cost for noninstitutional care. Further details are provided in exhibit 9.3.

EXHIBIT 9.3
Financial Impact of Institutional and Noninstitutional Long-Term Care

VA Geriatrics & Extended Care Services
Incurred Costs and # of Users During Fiscal Year 2017

Program	Incurred Cost (Billion $)	Users
INSTITUTIONAL LONG-TERM CARE		
Community Living Centers	3.78	42,680
Community Nursing Homes	0.88	30,670
State Veterans Homes	1.18	32,465
Subtotal Institutional Care	**6.44**	**106,083**
NONINSTITUTIONAL LONG-TERM CARE (NIC)		
Personal Care Services (HHHA, Community ADHC, Respite)	0.89	134,137
HBPC	0.67	54,893
Other (Purchased Skilled, Hospice, VA ADHC, SCI Home Care, Home Telehealth, CRC, MFH)	0.57	222,355
Subtotal Noninstitutional (NIC) Based Care	**2.10**	**354,323**
TOTAL VA PROVIDED GERIATRICS & EXTENDED CARE SERVICES	**8.58**	**414,658**
Any hospice/ palliative care (inpatient/outpatient)	0.65	22,261

Note: ADHC = Adult Day Health Care; CRC = Community Residential Care; HBPC = Home Based Primary Care; HHHA = Homemaker and Home Health Aide; MFH = Medical Foster Home; SCI = Spinal Cord Injury; VA = US Department of Veterans Affairs.

Source: Adapted from the US Department of Veterans Affairs.

Strategies

As VA strives to be a national leader in providing care for seniors, it must figure out how best to reduce healthcare costs. Its main options include the following:

- *Reduce or restrict services.* Ration who gets care, or what care they get.
- *Share costs.* Increase copayment; shift costs.
- *Reduce cost of services.* Lower salaries.
- *Meet care needs in a more efficient, lower-cost manner.* Avoid unnecessary costs by (1) preventing avoidable hospital days; (2) improving emergency care of frail older veterans; (3) optimizing nursing home utilization; (4) minimizing unnecessary procedures, duplication, and errors; and (5) aligning care with veteran and family goals.

VHA has implemented four strategies to overcome the public health challenges associated with the aging population: (1) targeting, (2) training, (3) teams, and (4) technology.

Targeting

VHA is targeting high-need, high-risk patients and aligning the intensity of its services with the wishes of the veterans being served. Risk stratification and targeting, along with point-of-care diagnostics and geographic information systems, can help create a data infrastructure to help veterans more efficiently. One tool that helps identify veterans at elevated risk of long-term institutionalization is the JEN Frailty Index, which provides a risk score, with levels 0 to 13, based on a count of 13 impairment categories identified from International Classification of Diseases diagnoses. Approximately 1,800 diagnoses codes are collapsed into the 13 categories (Kinosian et al. 2018).

Training

VA's second strategy involves increasing the number of geriatric-trained practitioners and caregivers in the workforce. As documented by the American Geriatrics Society (2019) and other sources (Cantor 2017), the current numbers are inadequate. One useful vehicle for training is Project ECHO (Extension for Community Healthcare Outcomes), a collaborative learning model in which experts connect via technology to providers who need training or support in problem solving (Project ECHO 2019). Another approach is to train caregivers so that they can better maintain the veterans at home (Hung et al. 2014; Zhou et al. 2016).

Teams

VHA can approach veteran senior care more holistically by creating interdisciplinary teams, using advanced care-delivery models, and emphasizing coordination of care, staff training, and caregiver support. VA has invested in several laboratories that develop and study the implementation of team-based approaches to care (Yano et al. 2014).

Technology

VHA is using technological approaches, such as telehealth, to provide care for veterans who live in remote areas. Such approaches can allow for the delivery of care without the need to travel great distances to a VHA facility (Atkins and Clancy 2017). Geriatric Research, Education, and Clinical Centers (GRECCs) in urban settings, for instance, provide expert consultation to veterans and to providers through the GRECC Connect program. Home telehealth for chronic disease management can expand the reach of VHA with services veterans want, helping to increase satisfaction, provide efficient care, and achieve good clinical outcomes (Hung et al. 2014).

Shifting from a Hospital Focus to a Home-Based Orientation

The VHA healthcare system evolved from a hospital-based model. Since 2000, with the implementation of the Millennium Bill, VHA has developed its clinic capacity, but some fundamental functions are still primarily performed through hospital care.

A substantial—and growing—proportion of veterans and their families want the option of living at their home for as long as possible. However, roughly 50 percent of veterans living in nursing homes did not receive any noninstitutional care (i.e., home- and community-based personal care and support) in the 12 months prior to their nursing home placement. Recent initiatives from within the VHA have begun focusing on services to enable veterans to stay at home and not be institutionalized.

VHA must find the best pathways for developing more efficient home and community-based services and for improving access to them. The home- and community-based services currently available are not well integrated; they comprise a patchwork of solutions and programs that function together inefficiently. Leaders at VHA Medical Centers have reported reluctance to invest in increased home and community-based services, and current approaches to identifying which patients truly need these services lack precision.

Data from patient surveys indicate that seniors far prefer to remain in their own homes during their later years, as opposed to going into institutions. Caregivers, however, often have mixed reactions: They want to provide the most loving and personal care for their family member, but they also must contend with the physical, emotional, and financial strains of caregiving. VA is now investing in efforts to provide support to caregivers, recognizing their importance in veterans' health.

VA operates a national call center and provides subsidies to caregivers of veterans. These subsidies were initially only for the care of veterans whose service was after the September 11 terrorist attacks of 2001, but they were extended to all veterans under the 2018 MISSION Act.

A new office for the "Choose Home" initiative, reporting to the undersecretary for health, is poised to provide strategies to target populations who are at risk of nursing home placement, identify combinations of services that are most appropriate to various situations, streamline referrals, and provide longitudinal case management coordinated with community resources.

In addition, the Elizabeth Dole Center of Excellence for Veterans and Caregiver Research was established in 2018. The goals of the center are to pilot innovative interventions; to develop and validate quality outcome metrics; to determine optimal combinations of services; and to integrate findings for dissemination across the VA (VA 2019b). The pilot programs, not yet rolled out as of this writing, will create a caregiver-inclusive curriculum and change the incentives for Medical Centers, so that leadership of VA facilities will want to invest in home and community-based services.

Fundamentally changing the VA culture from a hospital orientation to home orientation has the potential to substantially reduce costs associated with healthcare. Exhibit 9.4 shows the VA strategy for optimizing the veteran and caregiver experience under the Choose Home model.

Jose Lopez and the Clinic in the Southwest

VHA has invested considerable resources to advance and expand the field of geriatrics, both by establishing new clinical programs and by promoting education and research. The 20 federally mandated GRECCs, located across the country, are committed to

EXHIBIT 9.4
Potential Framework for Choose Home Model Benefits

How VA Will Optimize the Veteran and Caregiver Experience in the Choose Home Model

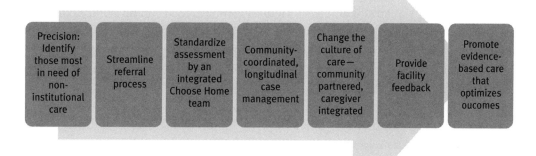

Source: Adapted from the US Department of Veterans Affairs.

research, education, and the development of novel clinical applications, and the Geriatrics and Extended Care Data and Analysis Center (GECDAC) supports VHA's data needs and evaluates the effectiveness and impact of its programs. GECDAC has also begun providing site-specific data to assist program development in settings such as the southwestern VHA clinic that Jose Lopez has begun managing. These VHA resources will be extremely useful as Jose tries to formulate a plan for serving the senior veterans in his region.

A Quality Discrepancy

A collaboration between the Providence VA Medical Center's Long-Term Services and Support Center of Innovation and GECDAC compared the quality of VHA-paid nursing homes and non-VA-paid nursing homes. Researchers found that the national average Star Rating for non-VHA-paid nursing homes was 3.25 (out of a maximum 5.00), whereas the average for VHA-paid nursing homes was only 3.00. 41.4 percent of VHA-paid facilities had only 1 or 2 stars.

In investigating why the VHA was contracting with lower-quality nursing homes, researchers found that, because operating under a VHA contract is burdensome on the institution, only nursing home facilities that needed to fill beds were doing so.

How should VA attempt to address this quality discrepancy between VHA-paid facilities and non-VHA-paid facilities?

Given that veterans aged 65 or older make up 60 percent of his clinic's enrolled clients, Jose suspects he can cut his budget significantly if he can improve the efficiency with which these veterans and their families are served. Jose's clinic is part of a Veterans Integrated Service Network (VISN), a regional VHA network, in the Southwest, and he reports to the director of an urban Medical Center. However, he cannot count on anyone in another unit to have the necessary depth of knowledge about senior services.

Jose outlines the tasks he needs to accomplish to come up with a plan for senior services that will apply to his clinic. He breaks his list into short-term and long-term actions. Tasks include the following:

1. Analyze the utilization data of his clinic to determine the extent to which senior veterans use expensive inpatient services, relative to national VHA benchmarks.
2. Determine how to identify senior veterans at high risk of needing expensive services, especially nursing home care. Given staff limitations, a highly detailed research tool is likely not practical. Assessment should take into account physical health status, mental health status, functional status, family/social support, and access to other community assets; all of these factors may be relevant.

3. Identify what data are needed to monitor the service use of senior veterans. This task involves gathering data from the array of services on the VHA continuum, many of which may not be located in his immediate community or operated by VHA.

4. Evaluate the potential value of adding a care coordinator position. This individual would be available to guide seniors in selecting the best level of care for their needs, help them transition across services, and enhance conditions to enable them to stay at home. The coordinator would also provide counseling and education to caregivers.

5. Assess the potential for using telehealth or other electronic systems to improve access to care and ongoing monitoring for senior veterans who live a significant distance from a VHA facility.

Questions

Fact and Data Analysis Questions

1. How is the word *veteran* defined? Who is eligible for VHA services?
2. Describe the organization of the US Department of Veterans Affairs and its subunits, including VHA.
3. What challenges does the aging of the veteran population pose for VA and VHA?
4. How are Medicare, Medicaid, and VHA related in the payment of health-related services for veterans aged 65 or older?
5. What challenges does the VHA face in attempting to switch from incentivizing hospital-oriented services to incentivizing home and community-based services? What can be done to counter these challenges?
6. What are VHA's options to reduce its healthcare costs? Which option is the most desirable and why?

Discussion Questions

1. Consider the priorities of Geriatrics and Extended Care: access, balance, and care coordination. Why are they important, and how do they help achieve the GEC's goals?
2. If you were a member of a VA hospital's leadership team, what information would you want before making any changes or rolling out a pilot program intended to improve the care available to older veterans?
3. VHA has numerous hospitals across the nation. What issues is it likely to face in implementing a new home care–oriented pilot program? What can be done to make the process smoother?

4. How can Jose make use of the GECDAC data and infrastructure despite not having extensive resources?

5. Assuming complete information about usage is necessary to maximize the efficiency of an aged veteran's care, what can a VHA clinic do to gather the essential information? How can the data be acquired from community service providers? What type of information system is appropriate and affordable for managing this information?

6. Jose made a list of tasks. What information or actions would be needed to complete each task?

References

American Geriatrics Society. 2019. "Where We Stand." Accessed June 27. www.americangeriatrics. org/where-we-stand.

Atkins, D., and C. M. Clancy. 2017. "Advancing High Performance in Veterans Affairs Health Care." *JAMA* 318 (19): 1927–28.

Beales, J. L., and T. Edes. 2009. "Veteran's Affairs Home Based Primary Care." *Clinics in Geriatric Medicine* 25 (1): 149–54, viii–ix.

Blackburn, J., J. L. Locher, M. A. Morrisey, D. J. Becker, and M. L. Kilgore. 2016. "The Effects of State-Level Expenditures for Home- and Community-Based Services on the Risk of Becoming a Long-Stay Nursing Home Resident After Hip Fracture." *Osteoporosis International* 27 (3): 953–61.

Cantor, M. D. 2017. "We Need More Geriatricians, Not More Primary Care Physicians." *NEJM Catalyst.* Published June 28. https://catalyst.nejm.org/need-more-geriatricians-primary-care/.

Clarke, P. M., R. Gregory, and J. A. Salomon. 2015. "Long-Term Disability Associated with War-Related Experience Among Vietnam Veterans: Retrospective Cohort Study." *Medical Care* 53 (5): 401–8.

DeCherrie, L. V., T. Soriano, and J. Hayashi. 2012. "Home-Based Primary Care: A Needed Primary-Care Model for Vulnerable Populations." *Mount Sinai Journal of Medicine* 79 (4): 425–32.

Eiken, S., K. Sredl, B. Burwell, and R. Woodward. 2017. *Medicaid Expenditures for Long-Term Services and Supports (LTSS) in FY 2015.* Published April 14. www.medicaid.gov/medicaid/ ltss/downloads/reports-and-evaluations/ltssexpendituresffy2015final.pdf.

Garrido, M. M., R. M. Allman, S. D. Pizer, J. L. Rudolph, K. S. Thomas, N. R. Sperber, C. H. Van Houtven, and A. B. Frakt. 2017. "Innovation in a Learning Health Care System: Veteran-Directed Home- and Community-Based Services." *Journal of the American Geriatrics Society* 65 (11): 2446–51.

Hung, W. W., M. Rossi, S. Thielke, T. Caprio, S. Barczi, B. J. Kramer, G. Kochersberger, K. S. Boockvar, A. Brody, and J. L. Howe. 2014. "A Multisite Geriatric Education Program for Rural Providers in the Veteran Health Care System (GRECC-Connect)." *Gerontology & Geriatrics Education* 35 (1): 23–40.

Kinosian, B., E. Stallard, and D. Wieland. 2007. "Projected Use of Long-Term-Care Services by Enrolled Veterans." *Gerontologist* 47 (3): 356–64.

Kinosian, B., D. Wieland, X. Gu, E. Stallard, C. S. Phibbs, and O. Intrator. 2018. "Validation of the JEN Frailty Index in the National Long-Term Care Survey Community Population: Identifying Functionally Impaired Older Adults from Claims Data." *BMC Health Services Research* 18 (1): 908.

Leff, B., C. M. Weston, S. Garrigues, K. Patel, and C. Ritchie. 2015. "Home-Based Primary Care Practices in the United States: Current State and Quality Improvement Approaches." *Journal of the American Geriatrics Society* 63 (5): 963–69.

Levy, C. R., F. Alemi, A. E. Williams, A. R. Williams, J. Wojtusiak, B. Sutton, P. Giang, E. Pracht, and L. Argyros. 2016. "Shared Homes as an Alternative to Nursing Home Care: Impact of VA's Medical Foster Home Program on Hospitalization." *Gerontologist* 56 (1): 62–71.

Levy, C., and E. A. Whitfield. 2016. "Medical Foster Homes: Can the Adult Foster Care Model Substitute for Nursing Home Care?" *Journal of the American Geriatrics Society* 64 (12): 2585–92.

Project ECHO. 2019. "About ECHO." Accessed June 27. https://echo.unm.edu/about-echo.

Reckrey, J. M., T. A. Soriano, C. R. Hernandez, L. V. DeCherrie, S. Chavez, M. Zhang, and K. Ornstein. 2015. "The Team Approach to Home-Based Primary Care: Restructuring Care to Meet Individual, Program, and System Needs." *Journal of the American Geriatrics Society* 63 (2): 358–64.

Segelman, M., O. Intrator, Y. Li, D. Mukamel, P. Veazie, and H. Temkin-Greener. 2017. "HCBS Spending and Nursing Home Admissions for 1915(c) Waiver Enrollees." *Journal of Aging & Social Policy* 29 (5): 395–412.

Thomas, K. S., and S. M. Allen. 2016. "Interagency Partnership to Deliver Veteran-Directed Home and Community-Based Services: Interviews with Aging and Disability Network Agency Personnel Regarding Their Experience with Partner Department of Veterans Affairs Medical Centers." *Journal of Rehabilitation Research and Development* 53 (5): 611–18.

US Department of Veterans Affairs (VA). 2019a. "Geriatrics and Extended Care." Updated February 18. www.va.gov/GERIATRICS/GEC_Leadership_And_Goals.asp.

———. 2019b. "The Elizabeth Dole Center of Excellence for Veteran and Caregiver Research." Accessed June 19. www.hsrd.research.va.gov/centers/dole/default.cfm.

———. 2019c. "VA Launches New Health Care Options Under MISSION Act." Published June 6. www.va.gov/opa/pressrel/pressrelease.cfm?id=5264.

———. 2019d. "Veteran Population." Updated May 24. www.va.gov/vetdata/veteran_population.asp.

———. 2019e. "Veterans Health Administration." Accessed February 27. www.va.gov/health/.

———. 2018a. "Geriatrics and Extended Care." Updated December 29. www.va.gov/GERIATRICS/Guide/LongTermCare/Home_and_Community_Based_Services.asp.

———. 2018b. "Veterans Health Administration: About VHA." Updated December 27. www.va.gov/health/aboutvha.asp.

———. 2016. "Geriatric Patient Aligned Care Team (GeriPACT)." Updated August 6. www.va.gov/GERIATRICS/Geriatric_Patient_Aligned_Care_Team.asp.

Vespa, J., D. M. Armstrong, and L. Medina. 2018. "Demographic Turning Points for the United States: Population Projections for 2020 to 2060." US Census Bureau. Published March. www.census.gov/content/dam/Census/library/publications/2018/demo/P25_1144.pdf.

VetPop16. 2017. *Veteran Population Projection Model 2016.* Washington, DC: Office of Enterprise Integration, Data Governance and Analytics, Predictive Analytics, and Actuary.

Yano, E. M., M. J. Bair, O. Carrasquillo, S. L. Krein, and L. V. Rubenstein. 2014. "Patient Aligned Care Teams (PACT): VA's Journey to Implement Patient-Centered Medical Homes." *Journal of General Internal Medicine* 29 (Suppl. 2): S547–49.

Zhou, C., A. Crawford, E. Serhal, P. Kurdyak, and S. Sockalingam. 2016. "The Impact of Project ECHO on Participant and Patient Outcomes: A Systematic Review." *Academic Medicine* 91 (10): 1439–61.

Useful Resources

- "Families Open Up Their Homes to Serve Veterans," by CBS News (www.cbsnews.com/video/families-open-up-their-home-and-hearts-to-serve-veterans/)
- National Center for Veterans Analysis and Statistics—Quick Facts (www.va.gov/vetdata/Quick_Facts.asp)
- US Department of Veterans Affairs—Geriatrics and Extended Care (www.va.gov/geriatrics/)
- US Department of Veterans Affairs—MISSION Act (https://missionact.va.gov/)
- US Department of Veterans Affairs—Veterans Health Administration (www.va.gov/health/)

10

FINANCIAL ANALYSIS: EVALUATING AN ANCHOR MISSION FOR CHICAGO'S NEAR WEST SIDE

Jason S. Turner

Case at a Glance

Overarching theme	The overarching theme of this case is the financial valuation of community health initiatives to a healthcare system.
Learning objectives	<ul><li>Articulate how to define a population.</li><li>Determine health disparities within a population.</li><li>Apply economic theories to reduce health disparities among populations defined by geography.</li><li>Calculate the direct financial impact of an anchor mission initiative on a sponsoring organization.</li><li>Evaluate the comprehensive impact of an anchor mission initiative on a given community.</li></ul>
Key terms	<ul><li>Anchor institution</li><li>Comprehensive return</li><li>Core business</li><li>Cost of capital</li><li>Direct impact</li><li>Ecological Model of Health</li><li>Net present value</li><li>RACI matrix</li><li>Social determinants of health</li><li>Social net present value</li><li>Time value of money</li></ul>
Management competencies	Financial analysis, population health management
Population/subgroup	Urban neighborhood
Health issue or condition	Multiple

Management Challenge

Rush University Medical Center (RUMC) is one of the largest healthcare organizations in the Chicago area, with hospitals in Oak Park, Aurora, and the Near West Side. RUMC is a not-for-profit organization that encompasses an academic medical center, multiple ambulatory sites, and a university singularly focused on training healthcare professionals (with a Medical College, a College of Nursing, a College of Health Sciences, and a Graduate College).

The institution has been an active community partner dating back to its early years. In 2016, RUMC changed its corporate mission from a focus on being "the best in patient care" to seeking to "improve the health" of the individuals and communities it serves (RUMC 2019). The evolution of its mission has allowed RUMC to approach health more holistically by engaging with the community via community health clinics, outreach and mentoring programs, and a variety of operational and community-based initiatives.

The charge to the executive leadership team is to explain to the board the impact of the past year's community-oriented activities on the hospital and on the community. Before committing resources to continue these community-focused initiatives, the board must be convinced that the investment of the health system's resources is worthwhile from the short- and long-term perspectives and that it benefits the community while not jeopardizing the financial or quality status of the health system.

Background

Consistent with its 2016 change in mission, RUMC adopted an "anchor institution" approach. The board understood this strategy to mean that RUMC would become a leading institution in serving the people in its geographic location, with its perspective expanding beyond healthcare to encompass the overall well-being of the community.

The impetus for the shift in mission can be linked to significant disparities in the health status and related conditions of Chicagoland neighborhoods. Social determinants of health (SDoH) factors (e.g., unemployment, job scarcity, poverty, environmental damage, violent crime) can vary substantially, even between neighborhoods that are nearly adjacent (Chicago Data Portal 2019). As a result, neighborhoods that are just a few stops from one another on Chicago's public transportation system can have enormous differences in life expectancy (see exhibit 10.1). West Garfield residents, for example, are expected to live to age 69, whereas residents living in the Loop (i.e., downtown Chicago) are expected to live to age 85 (RUMC 2017).

As an institution and in partnership with existing community-based organizations, collaboratives, and expertise, RUMC developed an anchor mission (AM) strategy to address the disparities and health needs identified on Chicago's West Side

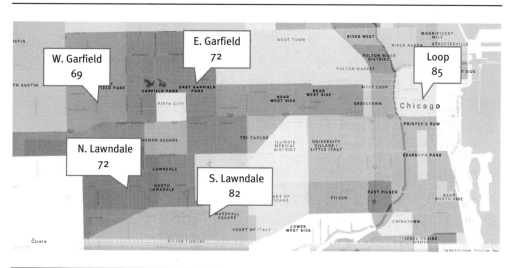

EXHIBIT 10.1
Life Expectancy
in Various
Chicagoland
Neighborhoods

Source: Used with permission from RUMC (2017).

and in adjacent communities. The overarching AM framework has the following aims (RUMC 2017):

- Improve social, economic, and structural determinants of health.
- Improve access to care and community resources.
- Improve mental and behavioral health.
- Prevent and reduce chronic disease.

Anchor Mission

Business unit leaders in key RUMC departments were asked to propose ways that their activities could support the community. The departments of human resources, supply chain/procurement, treasury/finance, capital projects, and community health equity identified levers of change under their control that could support the four AM aims. The results were mapped onto a 2×2 matrix with feasibility of the initiative on the horizontal axis and impact on the vertical axis (see exhibit 10.2). Initiatives that gravitated to the top and to the right provided initial indications of where RUMC should dedicate its efforts and resources.

The organization incorporated additional requirements that needed to be cleared before any activity could be integrated into a comprehensive RUMC anchor strategy. The initiatives should be targeted with the benefit intended for zip codes 60607, 60608, 60623, 60622, 60624, 60639, 60644, or 60651. The initiatives should have a comprehensive return rate of between 2 and 4 percent, and they should rank in the

EXHIBIT 10.2
Scalability and
Impact 2×2

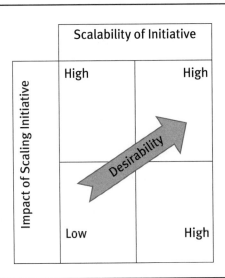

top two tiers of the Aeris impact and financial strength ratings. Aeris Insight is a financial information firm that specializes in providing data, consulting, and evaluation of investment in underserved people and places (Aeris 2019).

Business unit leaders, in conjunction with the RUMC CEO, the chief operating officer, the assistant vice president (human resources), and dedicated AM personnel, went further and developed a responsibility, accountability, consulting, and informing (RACI) matrix. The RACI matrix provided a means of developing an accountability structure with specific target measures and responsible parties, with regular reporting to the trustees. Ultimately, RUMC arrived at its first initiatives (see exhibit 10.3).

Economic Engine

In the previous year, RUMC generated more than $1.8 billion in revenue across the entire enterprise, of which $1.6 billion was related to the direct delivery of healthcare. As is typical for service industries, salaries and benefits were the largest component of the incurred expenses, accounting for $918 million. Additional purchased services accounted for $719 million.

To leverage the enterprise's significant economic engine, leaders proposed using the university and hospitals' supply chains as a means of supporting the anchor mission strategies. Specifically, RUMC explored hyperlocal procurement while also providing managers with the flexibility to source support services and goods from vendors in the identified zip codes. With the intermediate goal of increasing the number of new hires in AM communities through the shift in how RUMC is spending, internal progress was immediately measured by the following:

- The number of direct AM vendors doing business with RUMC
- The spending ($) associated with direct AM vendors

EXHIBIT 10.3
RUMC Change
Levers

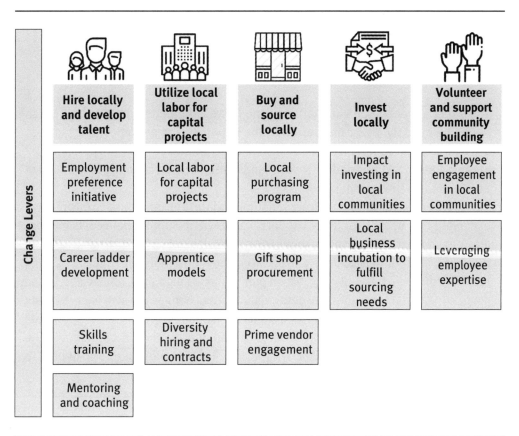

Source: Used with permission from RUMC (2017).

- The percentage of direct spending with AM vendors against the addressable spend
- The percentage of direct spending with AM vendors against total spend

Each of these metrics was established as a baseline in the first year of the strategy implementation and reassessed by RUMC leadership and the board of trustees.

Evaluation

The RUMC board of trustees is actively involved with the AM and understands that the evaluation of initiatives should be multifaceted and examined through more than one lens. If the anchor strategy is to maintain long-term viability, any losses incurred through the pursuit of an initiative must be subsidized by gains elsewhere in RUMC. As a result, the direct financial costs must be measured against direct financial benefits that accrue to RUMC. However, RUMC has also embraced a more comprehensive measure of return, which allows for consideration of benefits that accrue directly to the community and that only indirectly impact RUMC. For more information, see the accompanying text boxes.

Direct Impact Net Present Value (NPV) Formula

$$\text{Direct Impact NPV} = \sum_{t=0}^{\infty} \left(\frac{RUMC\ Benefits_t - RUMC\ Costs_t}{(1+r)^t} \right)$$

The direct impact is the summation of the RUMC's benefits minus costs in each period (commonly a year or quarter) of the initiative. The periodic impact is then discounted to account for the time value of money, where r is the firm's periodic cost of capital and t is the period. (Because funds require no discounting in the current period, $t = 0$ in the current period.)

When calculating the direct (and immediate) return, administrators have estimated that using hyperlocal vendors may drive up supply chain costs marginally (0–3 percent). The changes should not negatively affect satisfaction or quality measures, but they may positively affect facility pay-for-performance measures (e.g., readmission rates, hospital value-based purchasing adjustments, other value-based contracting tools) through social determinants. The changes are also likely to bring some improvements in the payer mix, a decline in bad debt, and some reputational benefits that come from advocating for and driving economic development in the community. On balance, the financial impact for RUMC is projected to be neutral to fractionally positive.

Comprehensive Impact NPV Formula

$$\text{Comprehensive Impact NPV} = \text{Direct Impact NPV} +$$

$$\sum_{t=0}^{\infty} \left(\frac{Community\ Benefits_t - Community\ Costs_t}{(1+s)^t} \right)$$

Evaluation of the comprehensive impact considers the benefits and costs that accrue to the community, not just to RUMC exclusively. The benefits may include increased employment rates, decreased poverty levels, reduced draw on state Medicaid funds, and the attraction of additional investment in the community. Although economic investment is generally positive, it does have the potential to drive gentrification of the area and displacement of the people the initiative is intended to support.

The comprehensive impact formula starts with the direct impact formula but adds the periodic benefits minus the costs that accrue to the community. Like the direct impact, the periodic impact must be discounted to account for the time value of money. The firm's cost of capital is used in the direct impact calculation but not in the community impact evaluation. Because the benefits accrue to the community (typically referred to as equity holders in a not-for-profit context where the hospital or system is viewed as a community asset), the cost of equity (s) is utilized (Wheeler and Clement 1990).

Interpretation of the direct and comprehensive impact formulae are the same as for traditional NPV formulae. If the summation of benefits minus costs (adjusted for time value of money) is positive, then the project generates value. If the summation is negative, the initiative destroys value and may require some subsidy. If a comprehensive evaluation has a negative NPV, the community benefits being derived from the initiative are not sufficient to warrant the cost, even though the community may not be bearing that full cost.

Charge to the Executive Leadership Team

The RUMC board of trustees and executive leadership team have confirmed that the programs comprising the anchor strategy cannot have a *direct* negative financial impact on the organization under the hyperlocal procurement and sourcing (direct impact NPV >= 0). However, the trustees have also requested an analysis of the financial impact on the community. To aid the analysis, the board recommends the use of data available through the Chicago Jobs Council (http://cjc.net/unemployment_data), City-Data (www.city-data.com), and the Chicago Data Portal (https://data.cityofchicago.org/) for baseline economic, employment, and population demographics (see exhibit 10.4).

The CEO gathers the other members of the executive team to set a due date and task outline to meet the request by the time of the next board meeting, two months from now.

West Garfield Park
Percent households below poverty: 40.3%
Percent unemployed: 25.2%
Per capita income: $10,951
Population: 27,582

East Garfield Park
Percent households below poverty: 39.7%
Percent unemployed: 16.4%
Per capita income: $13,596
Population: 34,249

Near West Side
Percent households below poverty: 21.6%
Percent unemployed: 10.7%
Per capita income: $41,488
Population: 74,850

EXHIBIT 10.4
Community
Data

Source: Data from Chicago Data Portal.

Questions

Fact and Data Analysis Questions

1. Based on the information provided, ignoring multiplicative impacts and assuming that 65 percent of the population is work eligible, determine the following:
   a. The immediate financial impact of increasing the per capita wages in each of the three identified communities (West Garfield Park, East Garfield Park, and Near West Side) by 1.5 percent
   b. The immediate financial impact of reducing unemployment by 1.5 percent in each of the three identified communities (assume individuals will be hired at the existing per capita income)

2. If RUMC invests $450 million per year in the local purchasing program and breaks even from a direct impact perspective, how large does the community employment impact need to be for the larger community to meet the 2.5 percent comprehensive return required to be included in the AM strategic plan? How much employment growth would be required if all of the efforts were focused on East and West Garfield Park?

3. Assuming that growing wages and employment requires time, calculate the financial impact of reducing unemployment for West and East Garfield Park if unemployment is reduced at .10 percent per year for the next eight years. For didactic purposes, assume wages and population remain unchanged and the community cost of equity (*s*) is .18 percent.

4. How would the comprehensive impact analysis be changed if the direct impact of the initiative were highly positive or highly negative?

5. In addition to the financial impact, what other ways might the RUMC anchor strategy affect the adults and children of the communities?

Discussion Questions

1. What other factors can be included in the evaluation of community impact?
   a. Based on your evaluation of the data sources provided, what factors would you include?
   b. How can other community improvements be put into the same financial language as the operational or direct impact?

2. What are the implications of changing how the population is defined? Should RUMC redefine the population based on disease state, age, income, or another factor?

3. Does a strongly positive comprehensive or community impact always outweigh operational losses (i.e., direct impact NPV that is negative)?

4. If the ultimate goal of the AM is to reduce health disparities, how does economic development work to improve social, economic, and structural determinants of health?

   a. Are there mechanisms that are more proximal/distal? Are those mechanisms related to the core competencies and business of RUMC?

   b. When should the board anticipate a decline in the disparities among the communities RUMC serves? Does that timing pose a challenge to the sustainability of the initiative?

References

Aeris. 2019. "About Aeris." Accessed July 1. www.aerisinsight.com/about/.

Chicago Data Portal. 2019. "Chicago Data Portal." Accessed July 1. https://data.cityofchicago.org/.

Rush University Medical Center (RUMC). 2019. "Mission, Vision and Values." Accessed July 1. www.rush.edu/about-us/about-rush-university-medical-center/mission-vision-and-values.

———. 2017. *Anchor Mission Playbook, Version 2.0.* Published June. www.rush.edu/sites/default/files/anchor-mission-playbook.pdf.

Wheeler, J. R., and J. P. Clement. 1990. "Capital Expenditure Decisions and the Role of the Not-for-Profit Hospital: An Application of a Social Goods Model." *Medical Care Review* 47 (4): 467–86.

Useful Resources

- *Gapenski's Fundamentals of Healthcare Finance* (Health Administration Press, 2018), by Kristin L. Reiter and Paula H. Song
- *Principles of Corporate Finance* (McGraw-Hill/Irwin, 2019), by Richard A. Brealey, Stewart C. Myers, and Franklin Allen

INFORMATION MANAGEMENT: CREATING A SYSTEM TO CARE FOR THE HOMELESS IN PHOENIX

Marisue Garganta

Note: This case describes programs initiated by Dignity Health St. Joseph's Hospital and Medical Center in Phoenix, Arizona. The specific scenario, however, was created for pedagogical purposes. The institutions involved assume no responsibility for the details as presented here.

Case at a Glance

Overarching theme	The case examines the information needed to manage the health status and utilization of a specific population group.
Learning objectives	• Delineate the information needed to manage the health of a specific population. • Examine issues involved in combining data from different data sets, including the sharing of data across organizations and across units within an organization. • Apply community health needs assessment data and metrics to programs for specific subpopulations within the community. • Evaluate evidence-based practices to improve the health status or health services utilization of a defined population. • Compile data to analyze the business case for a health organization to engage the community within a healthcare setting. • Measure the impact of organizational collaboration efforts on the health status of a community and its subpopulations.

Key terms	• Chronically homeless
	• Collective impact
	• Coordinated entry
	• Cross-sector collaboration
	• Hospital Readmissions Reduction Program (HRRP)
	• Hot-spotting
	• In-reach strategy
	• Interoperability
	• Medically Underserved Area (MUA)
	• Social determinants of health (SDoH)
Management competency	Information management
Population/subgroup	Adults experiencing homelessness
Health issue or condition	Multiple chronic health conditions

Management Challenge

The challenge facing the senior leaders of Dignity Health St. Joseph's Hospital and Medical Center (SJHMC) in Phoenix, Arizona, was how to manage a segment of the population that was having a major impact on the business operations of the medical center—adults who were chronically homeless—but for which essential data were not readily available. To provide quality care to this population over time while maintaining the financial integrity of the hospital's business would ultimately require a comprehensive information system encompassing data from a variety of different sources, including multiple community organizations.

Background

SJHMC's emergency department (ED) staff and medical center leadership teams had been challenged with the increased utilization by chronically ill and chronically homeless patients. According to Maricopa County and the Arizona Department of Health and Human Services, SJHMC had been the leading hospital in providing healthcare to the area's homeless population, despite the proximity of two other hospitals, including the county hospital. In 2015 and 2016, approximately 1,000 identified homeless patients frequented St. Joseph's ED, and the hospital expended nearly $9 million in "charity care." Homeless individuals often used the ED as their primary care provider and to help meet basic ongoing needs such as food or a place to rest. Some patients would come back multiple times throughout the day and night, especially if the weather was extremely hot or cold. SJHMC's most recent community health needs assessment had identified the homelessness issue as an unmet need.

To address the growing need to care for the homeless population, the medical center engaged its leadership and the community to develop new transitional care programs with an "in-reach strategy." Under this approach, nonprofits provide staff—such as community health workers, navigators, social workers, case managers, nurses, coaches, and peer mentors—to serve as part of hospital care teams and to assist patients transitioning from the hospital to the community, with support from community-based services.

Medical center leaders needed to be engaged in this process and, at times, provide additional financial resources to support the ongoing efforts. This new approach forced the healthcare executives to go "upstream" into the community context and to understand the impact of the community's social determinants of health on health status and healthcare utilization.

SJHMC led a community coalition to develop the organizational arrangements necessary for comprehensive attention to the needs of individuals and families who lack secure housing. Key to the organizational collaboration and short-term programmatic success would be an infrastructure of data to manage the program and the individual clients on a sustainable basis.

The CEO convened Jan, the vice president (VP) for nursing; William, the VP for finance; and Chan, the VP for information services, and charged them with developing a long-term plan for information system management that would accomplish the following:

- Identify patients at high risk of ED use or high risk of readmission because of the conditions of their housing
- Provide data to inform selection of evidence-based programs to improve the health of people experiencing homelessness
- Enable communication with patients who had no physical address, no phone, and no computer
- Track patients across multiple services within the health system, including use of the ED and multiple clinics and physician practices across the geographic service area
- Track service utilization across multiple community provider agencies
- Estimate costs of care from multiple organizations of different types, each with its own data system
- Identify "hot spots" in the community where the threat of homelessness and other social determinants of health put residents at risk of having poor health status or needing healthcare services
- Determine the health system's optimum business approach to issues of homelessness and high-risk SDoH, including the implications for the hospital's community benefit requirements

Jan, William, and Chan quickly concluded that this would be a major task! Moreover, the data needed for the various issues might overlap with regard to answering the business questions, but the sources of information were discrete. A long-range plan for information system management should be the goal.

About Phoenix and Maricopa County

With an estimated population of 4 million and growing, Maricopa County is the fourth most populous county in the United States. It is home to well over half of Arizona's residents. The county encompasses 9,224 square miles and includes 27 cities and towns, as well as all or part of five sovereign American Indian reservations.

Maricopa County is ethnically and culturally diverse. According to the US Census Bureau (2016), it has more than 1.2 million Hispanics (30 percent of all residents), 216,000 African Americans (5.3 percent), 157,000 Asian Americans (3.8 percent), and 77,000 American Indians (1.9 percent). About 14 percent of the population does not have a high school diploma, and 17 percent is living below the federal poverty level. More than 600,000 residents are uninsured (PolicyMap 2019).

The city of Phoenix, Maricopa's county seat, is the fifth largest US city by population and the most populous state capital. In 2017, its population was 1,626,078, with a median age of 33.3. Phoenix's surrounding communities include Tempe, Scottsdale, Glendale, Peoria, Tolleson, Avondale, Buckeye, Goodyear, Surprise, and Gila Bend. The Phoenix area is primarily served by SJHMC for acute care and trauma services. Exhibit 11.1 lists demographic and economic areas for SJHMC's primary service area, Maricopa County, and Arizona as a whole.

About St. Joseph's Hospital and Medical Center

SJHMC is part of Dignity Health, a San Francisco–based nonprofit healthcare system. With more than 60,000 caregivers and staff who provide care to diverse communities in 21 states, Dignity Health is the fifth largest health system in the nation. Dignity Health is member of Catholic Health Association (CHA), which has been a leader in community benefit services for decades (CHA 2019).

Founded in 1895 by the Sisters of Mercy, SJHMC is a 586-bed, not-for-profit medical center located in the heart of Phoenix. As of 2017, SJHMC had 4,565 staff members, 200 research employees, 183 employed faculty physicians, 1,109 credentialed community physicians, 260 residents in 20 specialties, and 813 volunteers (SJHMC 2017).

SJHMC provides a wide range of health, social, and support services, with special attention to the poor and underserved. The organization's mission, vision, and values (see exhibit 11.2) express a commitment to high-quality healthcare, advocacy, and collaboration with others in the community.

	SJHMC Primary Service Area	Maricopa County	Arizona
Population (estimated 2016)	2,902,805	4,088,549	6,728,577
Gender			
• Male	49.8%	49.5%	49.7%
• Female	50.2%	50.5%	50.3%
Age			
• 0 to 9 years	14.5%	13.8%	13.3%
• 10 to 19 years	14.2%	13.8%	13.6%
• 20 to 34 years	23.1%	21.2%	20.5%
• 35 to 64 years	36.0%	37.3%	36.7%
• 65 to 84 years	10.8%	8.0%	9.2%
• 85 years or older	1.4%	5.9%	6.7%
Race			
• White	47.4%	56.9%	77.8%
• Asian/Pacific Islander	3.6%	4.0%	3.2%
• Black or African American	6.0%	5.0%	4.3%
• American Indian/Alaska Native	1.7%	1.5%	4.4%
• Other/unknown	2.3%	2.3%	7.0%
Ethnicity			
• Hispanic	39.0%	30.3%	30.5%
Median income	$48,600	$53,694	$51,340
Uninsured	16.3%	13.9%	13.6%
Unemployment	4.8%	4.4%	5.4%
No high school diploma	17.2%	14.0%	13.8%
% of population 5+ non-English speaking	7.6%	9.2%	8.9%
Renters	44.4%	39.0%	36.9%
CNI score	4.0	3.4	
Medically underserved area	Yes		

EXHIBIT 11.1
Demographic and Economic Indicators

Note: CNI = Community Need Index.

Source: Compiled by Dignity Health St. Joseph's Hospital and Medical Center; data from US Census Bureau (2018).

EXHIBIT 11.2
Mission, Vision,
and Values of
Dignity Health
St. Joseph's
Hospital and
Medical Center

Mission

We are committed to furthering the healing ministry of Jesus. We dedicate our resources to:

- Delivering compassionate, high-quality, affordable health services;
- Serving and advocating for our sisters and brothers who are poor and disenfranchised; and
- Partnering with others in the community to improve the quality of life.

Vision

A vibrant, national health care system known for service, chosen for clinical excellence, standing in partnership with patients, employees, and physicians to improve the health of all communities served.

Values

Dignity Health is committed to providing high-quality, affordable healthcare to the communities we serve. Above all else we value:

- *Dignity*—Respecting the inherent value and worth of each person.
- *Collaboration*—Working together with people who support common values and vision to achieve shared goals.
- *Justice*—Advocating for social change and acting in ways that promote respect for all persons.
- *Stewardship*—Cultivating the resources entrusted to us to promote healing and wholeness.
- *Excellence*—Exceeding expectations through teamwork and innovation.

Source: Dignity Health St. Joseph's Hospital and Medical Center (2017).

SJHMC is a nationally recognized center for quality tertiary care, medical education, and research. It includes the internationally renowned Barrow Neurological Institute, the Heart and Lung Institute, the University of Arizona Cancer Center at St. Joseph's, and a Level 1 Trauma Center verified by the American College of Surgeons.

SJHMC draws populations from Maricopa County, from outside Maricopa County but within Arizona, and from outside the state. Its primary service area covers a defined geographic area surrounding the medical center, in the heart of Phoenix, and it does not exclude low-income or underserved populations. The primary service area is within the urban inner-city areas, though SJHMC also serves the suburban and rural communities for high-risk services. According to the Community Need Index (CNI), a proprietary tool developed by Dignity Health (2019), SJHMC's primary service area includes both moderate- and high-risk zip codes with significant socioeconomic barriers, including the threat of homelessness (see exhibit 11.3).

SJHMC's ED has a daily average of 85 visits. The payer mix has shifted slightly over the past five years but is still heavily weighted toward Medicaid (39 percent) and Medicare (28 percent). Commercial insurance (22 percent) and other payers (11 percent) make up the balance. In fiscal year 2018, SJHMC provided $188,681,867 in

EXHIBIT 11.3
Community
Need Index Map
with Zip Code
Areas

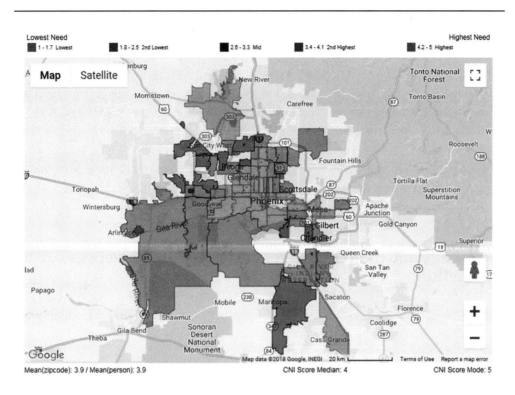

Lowest Need | Highest Need
■ 1 - 1.7 Lowest ■ 1.8 - 2.5 2nd Lowest ■ 2.6 - 3.3 Mid ■ 3.4 - 4.1 2nd Highest ■ 4.2 - 5 Highest

Mean(zipcode): 3.9 / Mean(person): 3.9   CNI Score Median: 4   CNI Score Mode: 5

Source: Reprinted with permission from Dignity Health St. Joseph's Hospital and Medical Center.

patient financial assistance, unreimbursed costs of Medicaid, community health improvement services, and other community benefits. The hospital also incurred $137,358,031 in unreimbursed costs of caring for patients covered by Medicare.

Community Need Index

The Community Need Index (CNI), developed by Dignity Health in 2004, is an analytical tool to identify high-needs areas within a health system's total service area. Dignity Health partnered with Truven Health Analytics to create a real-time database showing the economic and social characteristics of each zip code within a hospital's primary and secondary service areas.

The tool is updated annually and made available to all hospitals within the Dignity Health system to guide selection of programs. Underlying the data elements is the Dignity Health mission of providing care to the underserved and underprivileged members of its community. The CNI predated the now-widespread recognition by healthcare organizations that SDoH have a critical impact on the health of any individual.

Personal Perspective

Mr. SJ, fondly known as "Mr. 280," visited the hospital ED 280 times over a span of three years. He was never admitted, but he was seen multiple times in any given week. The only time the hospital staff did not see him was when he was in jail, during which time the clinical staff was left wondering if he was still alive. After reviewing Mr. SJ's case, the administrators of the ED decided a different approach was necessary. They decided to engage others in achieving a "big, hairy, audacious goal": finding Mr. SJ, stabilizing his health, and getting him housed.

A Strategy and Intervention for Caring for the Homeless Population

SJHMC was faced with an increase in the number of homeless patients utilizing the ED multiple times in one day. Many of these patients were seeking medical care, but many also sought a place to sleep, eat, and be safe.

SJHMC engaged multiple stakeholders to discuss the strengths, opportunities, aspirations, and results (SOAR) of meeting the growing needs of the homeless population. The leaders concluded that they needed to deploy the collective impact model to solve this complex problem (Collective Impact Forum 2014). Using this approach, the community health integration department at SJHMC moved away from working in isolation and in single partnerships toward a collectively engaged method of collaboration and problem solving.

Moving Toward Sustainable and Systematic Change

SJHMC embraced the collective impact framework to provide the structure with which to engage others to create sustainable and systematic change. Through this effort, SJHMC, in conjunction with the Corporation for Supportive Housing (CSH), helped launch the Frequent Users Systems Engagement (FUSE) initiative, with the aim of ending inappropriate overuse of emergency rooms, reducing inpatient hospitalization, and providing supportive services for chronically homeless individuals who are medically vulnerable. After two pilot initiatives, the FUSE model evolved into the Health and Housing of Medically Vulnerable People (HOMeVP) program.

For the HOMeVP program, SJHMC partnered with CSH, Valley of the Sun United Way, Circle the City, Health Care for the Homeless, Human Services Campus, Native American Connections, Arizona Housing Inc., and Arizona Behavioral Health Corporation. The coalition piloted the transition of homeless patients from hospital to home, reducing the need for these patients to seek shelter within the hospital and increasing their ability to be healthy. The program included the following:

- A full-time community health navigator position at Circle the City, to guide homeless participants through the myriad health and human services, with funding for the position provided entirely by one of the partner organizations
- Ongoing care coordination with a personal case manager
- Access to supportive housing
- Mental health counseling, with the goal of reducing risky behaviors

The FUSE I Model

Communities have spent billions of dollars on services that merely bounce vulnerable people between crises. The FUSE model sought to break that cycle by increasing housing stability and reducing crisis service use. FUSE connected participants from the hospital to healthcare and supportive housing, as shown in exhibit 11.4. The primary objectives of the pilot project were the following:

- Deepen collaboration across hospitals, health centers, and housing and social service providers.
- Place 15 frequent users of systems into supportive housing over 12 months, provide housing supports and intensive services to stabilize the participants, and track them over 12 to 18 months.
- Demonstrate that the Maricopa County–specific model can be effective across a range of outcome areas.
- Develop a sustainable financing model to fund hospital in-reach and housing/service provision.
- Reduce costly, unnecessary utilization of hospitals and homeless shelters.

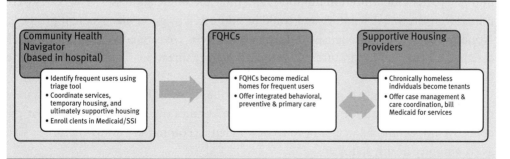

EXHIBIT 11.4
Homeless Community Health Navigation Flow

Note: FQHC = Federally Qualified Health Center; SSI = Supplemental Security Income.
Source: Homeless Community Health Navigation Flow: 2012, Corporation for Supportive Housing (CSH).

Information Management

Through FUSE and later HOMeVP, SJHMC was spearheading change in the way the medical center defined its role with patients and with other organizations in the community. Sustaining this change over time would depend on the ability to analyze what worked and what did not. This aspect called for a new approach to data and analytics, as well as to people and organizations.

Jan, William, and Chan—the three members of St. Joseph's C-suite charged with delineating the essential information management systems—first considered what they needed data for. They identified the following purposes:

- Identifying people coming to the ED and being admitted as inpatients who are currently experiencing homelessness or who are at risk of becoming homeless
- Tracking people who are experiencing homelessness across inpatient, ED, physician office, and other acute services
- Tracking people who are experiencing homelessness across use of services in the community
- Finding geographic areas in the community where residents are at high risk of homelessness (i.e., "hot-spotting")
- Measuring the collective impact of the community organizations partnering with SJHMC on the care of people experiencing homelessness
- Calculating the financial impact of the coordinated program on SJHMC, including the community benefit requirement

The team then made a list of all the organizations in the community that likely held data relevant to a given homeless client, including collaborative databases such as 211. Finally, the team considered the issues that they would need to address in identifying, securing, and managing the data from each unit within SJHMC and the community. These issues included interoperability, patient confidentiality, corporate propriety, multiple patient identification numbers, and multiple home addresses. The issues were primarily institutional in nature and could be addressed by good management practices. Nonetheless, the comprehensive information system envisioned, which would track clients over time and span internal and external organizations, would take time and resources to develop.

The team members presented a basic outline to the CEO for how such a system might be implemented for the future, if it were begun now. They concluded that the collective impact model would need to be applied to community infrastructure as well as community health status.

The Hospital Readmissions Reduction Program

Section 3025 of the Affordable Care Act (ACA) added a section 1886(q) to the Social Security Act establishing the Hospital Readmissions Reduction Program (HRRP). Effective October 1, 2012, the HRRP requires the Centers for Medicare & Medicaid Services (CMS) to reduce payments to hospitals that have excess readmissions, with the aim of making Americans' healthcare better by linking payment to the quality of hospital care (CMS 2019). Soon after the provisions went into effect, the Arizona Health Care Cost Containment System, the state's Medicaid agency, created similar and more imposing requirements that complemented the HRRP.

The potential for reduced payments and increased regulatory requirements created a fundamental change in the way care is provided both in and out of the hospital. The changes forced hospitals to work more closely with patients and caregivers, as well as with organizations and agencies within the community, on postdischarge planning. Hospitals were now being asked to identify individuals with frequent ED utilization, examine their length of stay within the hospital, and address their chronic health and social needs. The focus shifted away from "filling beds" and toward the need to keep people out of the hospital.

Leaders, both in government and in healthcare organizations, were forced to consider investing resources in cost-saving initiatives instead revenue-generating resources. With these changes, new and innovative initiatives sprang up to meet the ongoing needs of the community's most fragile members.

Questions

Fact and Data Analysis Questions

1. From what data sets will the team need to draw to compile a master data system for people experiencing homelessness?
2. How can you reach a client/patient who has no physical address, no post office box, no phone, and no access to a computer?
3. What are some of the technical issues involved in combining data sets across health and social service providers?
4. What would be the cost of creating a multi-institutional user data system?

Discussion Questions

1. SJHMC's goals for serving homeless patients are related primarily to the organization's mission and financial concerns. What would be the goals of some of the agencies with which it partnered?
2. Given the population of Phoenix, project the total number of people who might be experiencing homelessness at any given time. How many people would the collaborative need to reach to make a difference?
3. How could SJHMC and its coalition address the root causes underlying homelessness in addition to, or instead of, addressing homelessness once it happens to a person?
4. How do the health status characteristics of people experiencing homelessness affect their ability to change once they are in a stable housing situation?
5. What are the human issues involved in creating a multiuser data system?
6. Sketch out what a "client record" might look like for a homeless person who comes to the SJHMC ED but is also using multiple community services? What would the clinicians see? What would they record that those in community agencies might or might not see?
7. Some people are permanently homeless, whereas others are only temporarily without housing. How will these short-term clients be handled in a database designed to track people experiencing homelessness?
8. Some communities already have multi-institutional databases in place that record use of health and social services, such as 211 systems. What issues would SJHMC face in trying to combine existing multi-institutional information systems into the new system it is proposing for people experiencing homelessness?

References

Catholic Health Association (CHA). 2019. "Community Benefit Overview." Accessed July 2. www.chausa.org/communitybenefit/community-benefit.

Centers for Medicare & Medicaid Services (CMS). 2019. "Hospital Readmissions Reduction Program (HRRP)." Updated January 16. www.cms.gov/medicare/medicare-fee-for-service-payment/acuteinpatientpps/readmissions-reduction-program.html.

Collective Impact Forum. 2014. "What Is Collective Impact?" Accessed July 3, 2019. www.collectiveimpactforum.org/what-collective-impact.

Dignity Health. 2019. "Community Need Index." Accessed July 7. http://cni.chw-interactive.org/.

Dignity Health St. Joseph's Hospital and Medical Center (SJHMC). 2017. *St. Joseph's Hospital and Medical Center Community Benefit 2016 Report and 2017 Plan.* Accessed July 2, 2019. www.dignityhealth.org/-/media/cm/media/documents/Community-Benefit/2016-CB-St-Josephs-Arizona.ashx.

PolicyMap. 2019. "PolicyMap." Accessed July 7. www.policymap.com/maps.

US Census Bureau. 2018. "American Community Survey (ACS): 2013–2017 ACS 5-Year Estimates." Revised November 28. www.census.gov/programs-surveys/acs/technical-documentation/table-and-geography-changes/2017/5-year.html.

———. 2016. "Community Facts." Accessed July 2, 2019. https://factfinder.census.gov/faces/tableservices/jsf/pages/productview.xhtml?src=CF.

Useful Resources

- "Hospitals Invest in Housing for Homeless to Reduce ER Visits," by Pauline Bartolone, *Healthcare Finance*, October 2017 (www.healthcarefinancenews.com/news/hospitals-invest-housing-homeless-reduce-er-visits)

- "Housing Is a Prescription for Better Health," by Kathy Moses and Rachel Davis, *Health Affairs*, July 2015 (www.healthaffairs.org/do/10.1377/hblog20150722.049472/full)

- *Under the Safety Net: The Health and Social Welfare of the Homeless in the United States* (W. W. Norton, 1990), by Philip W. Brickner, Linda Keen Scharer, Barbara A. Conanan, Marianne Savarese, and Brian C. Scanlan (eds.)

- US Department of Housing and Urban Development—Point-in-Time Count resources (www.hudexchange.info/programs/hdx/guides/pit-hic/#general-pit-guides-and-tools)

- *Using Collective Impact to Bring Community Change* (Routledge, 2019), by Norman Walzer and Liz Weaver (eds.)

HEALTHCARE MANAGEMENT FUNCTIONS

This section offers cases that focus on the application of fundamental healthcare management functions to community-wide problems. Essential healthcare management functions have been defined in a variety of pedagogical models and parsed into competencies that incorporate both knowledge and the ability to apply that knowledge in practice.

Virtually all textbooks that present an overview of healthcare management list the following among the essential functions in which today's healthcare executives must be proficient:

- Organizational structure and behavior
- Strategic planning
- Marketing
- Finance and accounting
- Economics
- Information systems
- Quality assurance
- Law
- Ethics
- Human resources
- Communications
- Data analysis and analytical thinking

All of the cases in this book involve one or more of these functions as they apply to managing "beyond the walls" of a single health organization and across the boundaries of several organizations serving a given community or population segment. The cases in this section address specific healthcare management functions in greater depth than the cases in the other sections do.

In case 12, a community problem faced by a hospital—childhood asthma—is framed in terms of organizational ethics, and key decisions pertaining to community benefit and social determinants of health are underpinned by ethical deliberations.

Case 13, which deals with a continuing care retirement community, focuses on strategic planning and certain elements of marketing. Seeking to evolve from its previous insular, siloed approach, the facility tries to match contemporary market demand and better engage with the community.

Case 14 examines the challenges of physician recruitment and human resources management faced by a small critical access hospital as it tries to meet the immediate and long-term needs of rural constituents.

Case 15 involves the communications and marketing aspects of Live Well San Diego, a countywide effort by the San Diego County Department of Health and Human Services. The first task is to identify and characterize the multiple audiences involved with such an expansive initiative to improve the health of the county's population.

Finally, case 16 examines how multiple provider agencies can collaborate in a way that is sustainable over time to address the problem of HIV/AIDS resurgence. The case's focus on evaluating goals and means for sustaining community-wide collaboration makes it an appropriate final case for our discussion of population and community health.

ORGANIZATIONAL MISSION AND ETHICS: ETHICS AND POPULATION HEALTH IN GROVE CITY

Michael Rozier

Case at a Glance

Overarching theme	The focus of this case is on organizational ethics as they pertain to community and population health.
Learning objectives	• Identify the ethical issues related to managing population health. • Analyze the business case for a health organization to be involved with its community. • Contrast the financial implications of a new program's operating revenue/expenses with allocations to community benefit.
Key terms	• Belmont principles • Discernment • Distributive justice • Ethics • Nonprofit/not-for-profit organization • Organizational mission • Risk-based contract • Service area • Social determinants of health (SDoH) • Utilitarianism • Virtue ethics • Vision
Management competency	Ethics
Population/subgroup	Children
Health issue or condition	Asthma

Management Challenge

The leadership team of Greenville Hospital is determining how best to spend $100,000 that will be awarded by the local chamber of commerce for initiatives that benefit the community. Under one option, the hospital would implement a program to help children and families manage asthma and avoid hospital utilization. This new program could cause financial hardship for the hospital, however, because it would lead to decreased emergency room visits and hospital admissions. Other programs could be pursued that would benefit the community while not risking financial distress for the hospital. The number of children with severe asthma is particularly high in the hospital's service areas.

The members of the hospital's C-suite are debating the ethical issues of who will benefit from or be harmed by the hospital's ultimate decision. A secondary issue for management to consider is how to identify alternative cost-effective health promotion programs.

Background

Grove City is a metropolitan area of about 900,000 people that is experiencing a slight economic resurgence after decades of decline. Its city center comprises several historic neighborhoods, one of which is Greenville. Some of the city center neighborhoods are experiencing gentrification, whereas others still have pockets of deep poverty. About one-third of Grove City's population lives in the city center. The rest of the people live in suburbs and exurbs, which have higher average family incomes and better overall determinants of health. A summary of Grove City's demographic and economic indicators is provided in exhibit 12.1.

The historic neighborhood of Greenville contains several of the city's major cultural institutions, yet it also has very old housing stock, an underfunded school district, limited public transportation, and a scarcity of employment options that can provide a living wage. Most of the families living in Greenville have been there for several generations, and the neighborhood has a strong sense of community. One of the closed manufacturing plants in the area has been converted to an incinerator serving the entire city, and another is now a volunteer-run recreational center. The demographic and economic indicators of the Greenville neighborhood are different from those of other parts of Grove City.

Grove City's metropolitan area hosts four acute care hospitals. One of them, Greenville Hospital, is located in the city center and has its own emergency department. The other three hospitals are located in the city's suburbs, and two of these hospitals also have emergency departments. Several urgent care facilities are located outside the city center.

	Greenville Neighborhood	Grove City (excluding Greenville)	Grove City Exurbs
Total population	**95,647**	**615,831**	**110,520**
Race/ethnicity (%)			
White	25.2	76.1	81.0
African American	31.8	9.1	4.3
Hispanic/Latino	30.3	7.6	6.3
Asian	7.0	4.8	6.1
Other	5.7	2.4	2.3
Housing			
Total households	30,853	270,923	46,050
With children under 18 (%)	38.9	33.4	37.0
Renter-occupied (%)	55.8	25.4	20.1
Severe housing problems (%)	40.3	8.5	15.9
Economic			
High school graduation (%)	77.0	88.1	87.9
Unemployment (%)	9.6	4.5	4.5
Children in poverty (%)	27.4	12.0	14.1
Health			
Life expectancy	74.1	79.0	78.6
Low birth weight (%)	12.0	8.0	9.0
Adult obesity (%)	35.5	33.5	32.0
Adult smoking (%)	24.3	20.9	20.5
Uninsured (%)	11.6	7.3	8.5

EXHIBIT 12.1
Demographic and Economic Indicators

Note: Data are fictitious but constructed to resemble data for a real community.

Greenville Hospital and Its Mission

Greenville Hospital was founded in 1912. It is one of five acute care facilities in a regional nonprofit health system. The system has one other hospital in Grove City, in a southern suburb. The system recently invested significant resources to implement a single electronic health record across all its facilities.

As Grove City has grown, Greenville Hospital has remained the only acute care facility and the only emergency department in the city center. It has 250 inpatient beds, 205 of which are staffed. Occupancy typically runs about 40 percent, but the hospital feels compelled to keep specialty services open to serve emergency patients. The emergency department has a daily average of 85 visits. The payer mix has improved slightly over the past five years but is still heavily weighted to Medicaid (39 percent) and Medicare (28 percent). Commercial insurance (22 percent) and other payers (11 percent) make up the balance.

Greenville Hospital's financial health has improved slightly, in part because the surrounding neighborhoods have brought more residents with commercial insurance. Last year, it had its best operating margin (+.2 percent) in over a decade, and the outlook for the current fiscal year is similar. A positive bottom line is now occurring after many years of operating at a deficit (ranging from –.3 to –1.3 percent). Fortunately, the system's other hospitals have remained in strong financial health. The system also has a decent-sized and well-performing investment portfolio that has allowed it to cover the deficits of Greenville Hospital without hurting the other entities in the system.

Greenville Hospital provides a significant amount of uncompensated care. Over the past decade, the uncompensated care budget has averaged 9 percent of operating expenses. The equivalent of an additional 3 percent of operating expenses has gone toward a variety of projects characterized by the Internal Revenue Service (IRS) as community benefit.

The emergency department at Greenville Hospital has experienced a financial shift similar to that of the facility as a whole, from operating at a slight loss for many years to making a slight profit in the past two years.

Greenville Hospital and its parent system have always had a strong commitment to the people of Grove City. Even in the 1960s and 1970s, when the hospital was under major pressure to close because of financial concerns, the board of directors remained committed to maintaining a facility in the heart of the city. The organization's mission and vision have always provided a foundation for the organization's leadership and its employees (see exhibit 12.2).

An Intervention for Severe Childhood Asthma

A community coalition recently identified childhood asthma as one of the three biggest concerns for the Greenville neighborhood. When Greenville Hospital conducted its community health needs assessment (CHNA), as required by the IRS to maintain its tax-exempt status, asthma appeared as one of the community's "unmet needs." As a largely preventable condition primarily affecting impoverished children, asthma is a high-profile priority for community groups.

The new electronic health record system allows Greenville Hospital to easily identify those children who have had two or more visits to the emergency

EXHIBIT 12.2
Mission, Vision,
and Values
of Greenville
Hospital

Mission
To improve the health of the people and communities we serve and to manage illness with competence and compassion.

Vision
To be recognized for the quality of service we provide and our attention to patient care. We will continue to be the major health care provider in our primary service area of Grove City, as well as the hospital of choice for our medical staff. We recognize the importance of remaining a financially strong organization and will take the necessary actions to ensure that we can fulfill this vision for years to come.

Values
- Excellence—we deliver high-quality care, as understood by our patients and by external evaluation.
- Compassion—we remember that patients come to us at challenging moments in their lives, and we offer a loving response.
- Respect—we treat everyone we encounter with the equal dignity they deserve.
- Equity—we aim to reduce the health inequities present in our community.
- Collaboration—we work alongside our patients and others in our community to achieve our organization's goals.

department in the past year for severe asthma. This category includes 190 children, nearly all from the poorest census tracts in Greenville Hospital's service area. At least another 450 children under 17 live at the same addresses as the 190 children initially identified.

In keeping with the findings of the CHNA, the local chamber of commerce has made $100,000 available for a community health intervention. Raul, the president of the chamber of commerce, has indicated to the president of Greenville Hospital, Candace, that he thinks addressing childhood asthma would be an extremely worthwhile project. Based on previous interactions with Raul, Candace feels that he could be convinced to use the funds for a different project, but he would want a good justification for why it was not being used for asthma.

Candace meets with her leadership team. The director of community health, Gregory, is enthusiastic and says he knows of a highly effective program that has been shown to reduce the number of emergency room visits by almost 40 percent. The intervention involves a home assessment, appropriate home environmental remediation, and several home care check-ins.

Amal, the chief financial officer (CFO), believes the available funds can be used by Greenville Hospital in better ways. She indicates that an effective intervention for asthma, while good on many levels, would create significant financial pressures on the hospital because of the lost revenue from emergency room visits and hospital stays

Personal Perspective

Juliana is nine years old and lives with her father and her five-year-old brother. Her father works long hours. When Juliana's father is away, her aunt, who lives one block over, watches Juliana and her brother. Both Juliana's house and her aunt's house were built in the 1920s and are kept quite clean. However, they are both rentals, and the landlords have not invested in significant maintenance for many years, despite pleas from the tenants.

Juliana cannot remember a time when she did not have asthma. She has a mild attack about twice a week, but her inhaler really helps. She does not go anywhere without it. About once every four months, Juliana has an asthma attack that is much worse than usual. At first, she tries the inhaler, but she soon realizes the attack is not going away. She used to panic when these attacks happened, because she would feel like she was suffocating. Now she knows she has to find someone who can call an ambulance, which takes her to Greenville Hospital's emergency department. Either her dad or her aunt goes there with her. Sometimes she receives treatment and can go home later that day. Other times, she has to stay in the hospital overnight.

Juliana does not realize how many times she has come close to serious impairment because of her attacks. She also does not realize that the copayments for her inhalers are covered by the pharmaceutical company that produces them; otherwise, her family would not be able to afford them. Juliana's father and aunt are in a constant state of concern about her health, and they worry about what they would do if the pharmaceutical company discontinued the program that provides the inhaler. They are also concerned that Juliana's little brother will develop asthma, which, fortunately, has not yet happened.

(see exhibit 12.3). Amal does not advocate against the intervention, but she wants leadership to be aware that the funds could be directed in other ways that would either address diseases on which the hospital loses significant money or improve performance for some risk-based contracts.

Amal, like everyone in the room, wishes that the current reimbursement system aligned with doing good work such as asthma prevention, but she explains that "we just are not there yet." Unlike the programs in some other states, Greenville Hospital's state Medicaid program does not reimburse for home visits to address asthma.

Candace asks the leadership team to consider all the factors involved before returning for its next meeting, where the members will recommend either moving forward with the asthma-related program or looking for another priority area emerging from the CHNA that would both help the community and better protect the

EXHIBIT 12.3
Emergency
Department and
Intervention
Data

Greenville Hospital Childhood Asthma Data—Past Three Years

	Year 1	Year 2	Year 3
Utilization			
Number of ED visits for childhood asthma	620	587	603
Percentage of ED visits for childhood asthma that lead to hospitalization	17.4%	15.3%	17.0%
Average length of stay for asthma-related hospitalization (in days)	1.2	1.4	1.2
Percentage of those visits from children who would qualify for intervention	82%	85%	84%
Finances			
Average asthma-related ED reimbursement (across all payers)	$902	$913	$920
Average cost for asthma-related ED visit	$840	$855	$869
Average asthma-related hospitalization reimbursement (across all payers)	$3,020	$3,041	$3,080
Average cost for asthma-related hospitalization	$2,263	$2,400	$2,431

Notes: Data constructed to resemble figures for a real institution. ED = emergency department.

Asthma Data Projections for Home-Based Intervention

Cost of intervention:
- $610 per household
  - $110—initial assessment
  - $350—average cost of remediation actions
  - $75—follow-up visit (×2)

Effectiveness of intervention:
- 37% reduction of total visits
- 68% reduction of most severe visits that lead to hospitalization

organization's bottom line. Candace tasks the members of the leadership team with gathering specific information to report at the next meeting:

- Amal, the CFO, is asked to bring specific projections of the decrease in emergency department and admissions revenues that would occur if the new preventive program were successful, as well as the costs of the program, given case managers and home care. Greenville Hospital has no risk contracts that cover children, so fee-for-service can be assumed. Amal will need to make, and articulate, any other financial assumptions.

- Gregory, the director of community health, is asked to evaluate the hospital's last CHNA and determine whether any part of the outreach could be included on the IRS Form 990 Schedule H report, as part of the hospital's community benefit contribution. He is also asked to use the CHNA and work with Anna, the director of quality assurance, to identify other major health concerns and consider evidence-based interventions that might address those concerns. They will start by consulting the Community Guide, available online through the Centers for Disease Control and Prevention.

- Harvey, the chief information officer, is asked to explore whether the asthma concern could be addressed through a low-cost technological solution, such as a mobile application that could alert children or families before a major problem occurs. The app strategy could help Greenville Hospital improve its use of social media and mobile technology, showing the community and the rest of the health system that the hospital offers state-of-the-art care, despite its older facility and neighborhood.

- Shonda, the director of marketing, is asked to draft a communication strategy to use for the chamber of commerce funding. Candace would like to know whether the strategy would differ if the hospital went with the chamber's original recommendation of the asthma program or with a different program put forward by hospital leadership. Candace is concerned that a narrative could potentially emerge suggesting that the hospital used the funds to benefit its own bottom line rather than to address community priorities. Candace may also need to involve Gerard, the system's director of governmental relations, as any major community-level intervention would likely benefit from the support of local political leaders.

Select Ethical Principles

Candace knows that each member of her leadership team will consider the situation in a different way. At the same time, she wants to make sure that her leadership team is aware of the code of ethics for healthcare executives. She asks each member to review the Code of Ethics of the American College of Healthcare Executives—especially parts III and V, which pertain to responsibilities to the organization and responsibilities to community and society. In addition, Candace asks James, the pastor who coordinates the palliative care team, to provide the leadership team with basic information that can be applied when faced with ethical dilemmas. James describes the following ethical frameworks.

Utility

In its simplest form, utilitarianism asks which action will produce the greatest good for the greatest number of people. Some elements are easy to quantify. For example, determining how many hospital admissions will be prevented—and thus how many lost days of school for children or lost days of work for parents will be avoided—is a relatively straightforward calculation. Determining the effect of the program on the hospital's annual revenue can be similarly simple. However, quantifying the effect on the hospital's reputation of pursuing a plan other than the one recommended by the chamber of commerce becomes more difficult.

Despite the challenges, all quantifiable consequences must be calculated to determine which action brings about the greatest good for the greatest number of people. Cost-effectiveness comparisons rely on a utility-based ethical framework.

Virtue

Virtue ethics is a classic framework that has been in use since the time of Aristotle. Key questions ask: Who am I? Who do I want to be? How must I behave to get there? Or, from an organizational perspective, who are we? Who do we want to be? How must we behave to get there?

Virtue emphasizes that who you are influences what you do, and what you do shapes who you are. One might look at Greenville's mission, vision, and values and ask what decision the hospital should make if it is interested in being true to its values. Of course, values can conflict, and when that happens, the organization must decide which are most important. This hierarchy of values is often left unspoken or implicit, but ethical dilemmas can be ideal moments to make such a ranking explicit.

Virtue ethics is often unsatisfying for people seeking a clear answer to their ethical dilemma. However, compared to other frameworks, it can better reflect the nuance of individual and organizational behavior.

Distributive and Procedural Justice

Justice has at least a dozen different meanings, so the concept can be either extremely useful or extremely confusing. For this case, an important dimension is distributive justice, or the proper allocation of limited goods among a group of individuals.

The US healthcare system uses the principle of distributive justice to justify distribution to each person based on need (e.g., allowing people with disabilities, but not their nondisabled counterparts, to enroll in Medicaid), to each person equally (e.g., giving each eligible senior the same basic Medicare program), and to each according to social contribution (e.g., maintaining a health system for veterans). Even though these approaches employ different logics, and indeed might result in different allocations, each could be described as a "just" distribution.

Some ethics scholars claim that society will never be able to agree on what distribution is actually fair, so the process itself must be fair. Among other things, a just process would ensure that only relevant criteria are used in the decision process, that all stakeholders who are affected by the decision have a voice, and that the process is appropriately transparent. Justice is a noble end to pursue, but it is far more complex to administer than healthcare executives would like to admit.

Utility, virtue, and distributive and procedural justice are among the key ethical principles or frameworks that might be used in this case or in similar situations. Clinical ethics tends to rely on autonomy, beneficence, and justice, whereas public health often uses a human rights framework or arguments for sufficiency. As the work of population health identifies new financial, clinical, operational, and technological questions, new ethical questions will no doubt emerge.

Avoiding the Application of Medical Ethics to Community and Population Health

Discussions of ethics in healthcare are often governed by three ethical principles: autonomy, justice, and beneficence (which encompasses nonmaleficence). Collectively known as the Belmont principles, they are frequently used to negotiate dilemmas in clinical care and research. Autonomy—the ability of patients or research subjects to make informed decisions about their care—is the dominant principle, in large part because the historical roots of healthcare ethics were in response to situations in which patients and research subjects had been deceived or forced to take part in dangerous experiments (National Commission for the Protection of Human Subjects of Biomedical and Behavioral Research 1979).

The ethical questions related to community and population health, however, are different from the ethical questions of clinical care and research. The most important difference is that the object of analysis in community and population health is often an organization or an entire population, rather than an individual patient. Therefore, even though the ethical decisions take place in hospitals and health systems, the principles of medical ethics will rarely be the most appropriate. Ethical frameworks from the fields of organizational studies, public health, and community engagement are generally more useful when considering dilemmas in community and population health. These frameworks include virtue ethics, ethics of care, communitarian ethics, human rights, and many culturally specific concepts.

Key Points About Ethical Discernment

Ethical discernment is not an easy process. If a program decision presents an ethical dilemma, decision makers should be aware of the tension involved and work to see the situation from all possible angles. At the same time, a decision must be made, and it often must be justified in ethical terms. The following are some key points to keep in mind when confronted with a decision that has ethical implications.

First, identify the most important ethical question (or questions) that must be answered. One can easily become distracted by or focus too heavily on relatively minor aspects of a case. Clearly articulating the question at the center of the case—and ensuring that others would articulate it in the same way—can be extremely helpful.

Second, in today's world, good ethics requires good data. Ethical considerations should be grounded in the real world. Decision makers may need to determine the evidence pertaining to an intervention's effectiveness, assess the current regulatory environment, calculate the financial implications of a decision, and identify aspects of the case that cannot be known or are subject to significant probability. In the end, a good ethical discernment cannot take place without gathering the best possible data. Decision makers should be held accountable for obtaining current and comprehensive information pertaining to the decision.

Third, "ethics" should not be used merely to justify a foregone conclusion. When confronted with an ethical dilemma, most of us will have an instinctive response about what we think is correct. Understanding where these instincts come from can illuminate our personal ethical frameworks and biases. In healthcare, senior executives and board members must be open to starting with principles and allowing them to lead to a conclusion that might not have been initially favored. Ethical analysis should be as rigorous as financial analysis, and healthcare executives should be able to justify their ethical calculations as well as their financial calculations.

Personal Perspective

Candace, the chief executive of Greenville Hospital, has been with the system for over 20 years and has led the hospital for the past four. She is originally from Grove City, and she knows how vital Greenville Hospital is to the neighborhood.

Candace's husband is worried about her because she is always at work and often has to miss their children's events. Candace gets very little sleep and has recently had some mild anxiety attacks. Much of her stress comes from concerns about the stability of Greenville Hospital. The hospital has performed well in the past couple years, but Candace anticipates that a major disruption may be coming to healthcare in general, to the parent system, or to the hospital itself, which will risk peeling off the most profitable service lines. She is unsure whether the hospital or its parent system will have the wherewithal to survive the coming tumult.

Greenville Hospital is one of the most important employers in its area of the city, and Candace is greatly concerned about potential downsizing. The hospital currently runs a lean operation, but she knows that any deterioration in its financial position will likely mean more layoffs. Candace has worked hard to create a positive workplace culture, and she fears what downsizing might do to the image of the hospital in the community and the environment for employees at the organization.

Fourth, ethical discernment in a professional setting is most often a shared enterprise. Individual leaders are often the ones to ultimately make the decision, but the process of reaching that decision benefits from other voices. An organization might already have its own process for major ethical discernment, or perhaps now is the time for the organization to develop one. Having an established process helps ensure that all the voices that should be included actually are. This process is particularly important as we enter an era of community health. A shared process helps generate buy-in from people who disagree with the ultimate decision.

Moving Forward

When Greenville Hospital's leadership team reconvenes the following week, all the members report on the information they have gathered and present their own assessments of the ethical challenges of the situation. Candace leads the group through careful consideration of the data, as well as the ethical issues related to use of the $100,000.

What should the leadership team decide to do? How will they explain their decision to the executives at the system level, to the chamber of commerce, and to the community?

Questions

Fact and Data Analysis Questions

1. Consider the statistics of the Greenville neighborhood, and compare them with those of Grove City, using the data supplied. What additional data would be useful in analyzing the problem of asthma or potential solutions?
2. Compare the mission and core values of Greenville Hospital with those of a community hospital in your area. Does not-for-profit or for-profit status matter?
3. Explore the condition of asthma, including its prevalence and incidence in your area, its impact on children, and average annual costs for care.
4. Calculate the financial implications to the health system of revenues from emergency department visits and inpatient admissions of children with asthma.
5. What other programs to ameliorate asthma can be implemented in a community such as Grove City? What evidence is available to support their likely success?
6. What measures could be used to evaluate the success of a community-oriented program to ameliorate asthma?

Discussion Questions

1. If you were Candace, how would you frame the central question for your leadership team? Summarize the dilemma in a single sentence.

2. If you were a member of the leadership team, what additional information would you want as you considered the question at hand? (Students can form teams, and each person can take one of the C-suite roles. They can gather the requested information, prepare an initial ethical assessment, and bring their findings to the following week's discussion.)

3. Who should be involved in making this decision? How transparent should the organization be with its own members, with the funder, and with the community as to what factors were considered in making the decision?

4. What is the role of the board in making decisions about new programs such as the asthma initiative?

5. What ethical principles are most relevant to this case? To what conclusion do those principles lead?

6. How would an increase in risk-based contracting change the challenges faced by the leadership of Greenville Hospital?

7. What other situations related to community or population health have a major ethical dimension at their core? What is the central ethical question in each situation? How do ethics pertaining to community health differ from ethics pertaining to the health of individuals?

8. What role should ethics play in the business decisions of complex organizations such as hospitals and health systems?

9. If the asthma intervention were more effective or less effective, how might management's final decision be affected? If the financial position of Greenville Hospital were better or worse than it currently is, how might management's ultimate decision be affected?

10. How can governance structures, such as boards of directors, incorporate attention to ethics in their work?

11. With what other organizations in the community might Greenville Hospital partner to use the $100,000 most effectively to improve the asthma problem for the future?

Reference

National Commission for the Protection of Human Subjects of Biomedical and Behavioral Research. 1979. "The Belmont Report." US Department of Health and Human Services. Accessed July 9, 2019. www.hhs.gov/ohrp/regulations-and-policy/belmont-report/read-the-belmont-report/index.html.

Useful Resources

- American College of Healthcare Executives—Code of Ethics (www.ache.org/abt_ache/code.cfm)
- The Hastings Center—Health and Health Care (www.thehastingscenter.org/our-issues/health-and-health-care/)
- Healthcare Cost and Utilization Project Statistical Brief: *Trends in Pediatric and Adult Hospital Stays for Asthma, 2000–2010* (www.hcup-us.ahrq.gov/reports/statbriefs/sb169-Asthma-Trends-Hospital-Stays.pdf)
- The Community Guide (www.thecommunityguide.org)

13

LONG-TERM CARE: DEVELOPING A STRATEGIC PLAN FOR EVERGREEN CONTINUING CARE RETIREMENT COMMUNITY

Robert E. Burke

Overarching theme	The overarching theme of this case is the application of principles of strategic planning and marketing to help a long-term care institution transition from its insular past into a future enmeshed in its community.
Learning objectives	<ul><li>Outline the elements of a strategic plan.</li><li>Analyze a target audience.</li><li>Apply concepts of marketing to evaluate a product.</li><li>Define *long-term care*.</li><li>Identify trends and attitudes toward long-term care for seniors.</li><li>Delineate the elements of a community's healthcare system, including those related to long-term care.</li><li>Explain the rationale for and the components of a continuum of care.</li><li>Evaluate the workforce providing long-term care services.</li><li>Differentiate the financial management of long-term care from that of acute care, including the application of population health management.</li><li>Apply business principles to institutions engaged in long-term care, including principles about the role of governance.</li></ul>
Key terms	<ul><li>Assisted living</li><li>Continuing care retirement community (CCRC)</li><li>Continuum of care</li><li>Independent living</li><li>Long-term care</li></ul>

- Marketing
- Medicaid
- Medicare
- Medicare Managed Care
- Post-acute care
- Skilled nursing faculty (SNF)
- Strategic planning

Management competencies	Strategic planning, marketing
Population/subgroup	Seniors
Health issue or condition	Long-term care

Management Challenge

The management challenge of this case is to develop a strategic plan for a continuing care retirement community (CCRC). CCRCs are multilevel, self-contained communities that provide various services for individuals as they age and as their needs change.

The board of Evergreen Continuing Care Retirement Community (ECCRC) has awarded your consulting firm a contract to prepare a strategic plan to position the organization for the future. The board realizes that the market demand by consumers for CCRCs has changed significantly. Greater emphasis is now placed on integration into the community, rather than separation, which creates challenges for the institution, its structure, and the way it delivers a range of services. Further complicating matters are the ongoing changes in the workforce that provides services for ECCRC. In short, Evergreen needs to become better integrated with the community, its seniors, its workforce, and its health and support systems.

Because many Americans do not fully understand or plan for long-term care, selling a "product" that addresses the demand for such care can be a challenge. Nonetheless, a tsunami of demand for the services needed in old age is expected with the aging of the baby boom generation (i.e., people born between 1946 and 1964). The ECCRC board is concerned that the product for the future must be designed now, and its implementation and marketing planned as well.

Background

The senior staff of ECCRC and its C-suite are working at 100 percent of their capacity to ensure the safe operation of the facility. They are, perhaps, too invested in the current model of service and financing to actively envision change for the future. The

What Is a Continuing Care Retirement Community?

A continuing care retirement community, also known as a life care community, offers older adults an array of residential and support services at a single geographic site, in combination with predetermined financial arrangements.

The CCRC concept became prevalent in the United States in the late 1960s and the 1970s. Typically, an individual or couple would move into a community and make a substantial financial commitment, and the community would guarantee to make available whatever services were needed to maintain the individual or couple's health throughout the remainder of their life.

Financial arrangements have included a large initial buy-in fee and monthly payments. The monthly payments might be increased if service intensity needs to increase as a result of deteriorating health status. Residential options have included independent living in freestanding houses or apartments, assisted living, and skilled nursing facilities. Support services have included on-site health clinics, home health care, transportation, social events, and the availability of laundry, food preparation, and housekeeping.

The early models of CCRCs had a tendency to overcommit in terms of the services delivered, and many used inaccurate actuarial models. Many CCRCs went bankrupt as a result. These developments forced a change in the financing approaches used by the industry, bolstered or mandated by state regulations.

Over the past few decades, CCRCs have changed both their financial models and their service models to reflect seniors' changing preferences. Nonetheless, the "product" of a CCRC has become less appealing to the current cohort of seniors than to those of past generations.

board, therefore, has proposed that the CEO hire a consulting firm to perform a market analysis of ECCRC's current product and to develop a new strategic plan.

The consulting firm must take the concepts of population and community health and apply them to long-term care. The firm will report to the CEO, and the board will review the firm's analysis and use it as a basis for decisions regarding Evergreen's future.

The new strategic plan is to be divided into two time frames: between now and 2026 and between 2027 and 2046. The board expects the consulting firm to develop two scenarios, one for each time frame, that will sustain the mission of ECCRC and ensure its financial viability. The board has requested that the strategic plan have six sections:

1. Population and demographics, including trends in attitudes
2. Market positioning, product definition, product life cycle, and competition

3. Finance and payment
4. Workforce availability and capability
5. Continuum-of-care systems and partners
6. Visibility and community awareness

   Key management elements include the role of the board; the mission, vision, and values of the institution; clearly articulated goals and SMART objectives (i.e., objectives that are specific, measurable, attainable, relevant, and time bound); marketing concepts, such as product life cycle and product expansion; and the strategic planning process. Content issues include long-term care, the continuum of care, collaboration among community agencies, case management, workforce characteristics, and the financing of long-term care.

   The board has chosen your consulting firm for this task, because your staff are experts in the history, payment, policies, and operating nuances of the continuum of long-term care.

The History and Context of Evergreen Continuing Care Retirement Community

Evergreen is in a far suburb of a metropolitan area. The metropolitan area has a population of about 5 million, and the county in which ECCRC is based has a population of a little over 1 million. Exhibit 13.1 provides relevant demographic data for the county. The demographics are changing in terms of age distribution, immigration and language status, education, and income.

EXHIBIT 13.1
Demographic Data for the County

Age	2015	% Distribution	2025	% Distribution
0–44	606,550	59%	637,210	60%
45–64	285,790	28%	227,120	21%
65+	143,660	14%	195,680	18%
Total	1,036,000	100%	1,060,010	100%

Race/Ethnicity	2015	% Distribution	2025	% Distribution
White	93,139	65%	105,565	55%
Black	17,142	12%	27,595	14%
Hispanic	10,814	8%	20,478	11%
Other	22,226	16%	38,428	20%
Total	143,321	100%	192,066	100%

(continued)

Financial Indicator	2015	2025
Median income	120,974	80,945
Median home price	207,300	300,000

Annual Migration into or out of County				
Age	In	% of Pop.	Out	% of Pop.
Age 65–69	1,168	2.70%	1,215	2.80%
Age 70–74	1,006	2.70%	887	2.90%
Age 75+	1,989	3.30%	1,108	1.90%
Total	4,163	3.10%	3,210	2.40%

EXHIBIT 13.1
Demographic
Data for the
County
(continued)

Source: Extracted from sample census data.

Evergreen was the first CCRC in the county. Over the past 100 years, the organization has evolved from a rural, religious-based old-age home to a multilevel CCRC operated as a nonprofit organization. The expansion of CCRCs for this suburban region is governed by certificate-of-need regulations and state licensing laws. The financing of CCRCs is also governed by the state.

Today, ECCRC has a large geographic area, but it is land-locked, surrounded by urban expansion. The complex has three distinct levels of care: independent living, assisted living, and skilled nursing. Although Evergreen's mission, vision, and values are based in its religious roots, the organization is freestanding and does not rely on any religious organization for current or future funding.

Over the past decade, the percentage of occupied units at ECCRC has fallen, most dramatically in the independent living units. One explanation for this trend is that a decline in the value of real estate, both locally and nationally, has made it difficult for new residents to use proceeds from the sale of a home to pay the CCRC entry fee.

Another explanation is that ECCRC has lost some market share to newer types of organizations that are perceived by the public to be more modern and to offer more of what clients and their families want. Some of these emerging organizations have changed their financing model to a straight rental contract, as opposed to ECCRC's long-standing model of an entry fee plus a monthly rental fee. An additional model is a health insurance policy that includes supplemental services arranged with providers throughout the community.

The way Evergreen delivers its services might also be a concern. Because of its classic old-age home beginnings, the organization is more comfortable offering services within its own "brick and mortar" buildings than developing community-based services to be delivered directly to clients in their own homes. In addition, with its long history as a freestanding organization, ECCRC has no experience in developing and running services that are shared among several providers. Current trends in quality and consumer preference indicate that seniors would rather remain in their own homes and have services orchestrated around them than go to a place where services are readily available and centralized. Families, too, seem to prefer care at home to care that is considered "institutional" in nature.

Personal Perspective

William is 87 years old. Ellen, his wife of 60 years, passed away a year ago. William has been living in the home that the couple purchased 27 years ago, when they "down-sized" from raising their family and both retired from work. After 27 years, William and Ellen had accumulated a lot of stuff! The house holds a lot of special memories.

William is perfectly content with his housing arrangement. He has a lot of friends nearby and finds his local community to be a comfortable and active place to live. William's children, however, are trying to persuade him to move—either near one of them or to a CCRC. The children are concerned that, should William become ill, he could become stranded with no one to take care of him.

William definitely does not want to move halfway across the country, especially to a cold climate that would be inhospitable to his golf game. He assures his children that he knows a lot of local service agencies, including those that he called upon when his wife was ill. Still, to appease his children, he visits a local CCRC that has an excellent reputation. He tours the physical plant, finds lunch reasonable, and examines the financial terms. He is not convinced that a CCRC is for him!

The board of ECCRC, in executing its fiduciary duty, knows that it must take definitive action to ensure that the organization's mission is not threatened by a lack of planning or even bankruptcy. The organization therefore must adapt its product to the market.

Addressing the two time frames is critical. The first period, in the immediate future, has the existing buildings but a relative shortage of potential clients—as indicated by ECCRC's vacancy rates between 15 and 10 percent. The second period, however, has the potential "silver tsunami" of baby boomer clients. These individuals might not want the traditional services currently being offered by ECCRC, but they will be seeking some type of long-term care for many years to come.

Evergreen's management realizes that it needs to get a handle on the way residents of the local area are thinking about their long-term care options. Last year, the CEO hired a professional group to run two focus groups, the findings of which are summarized in exhibit 13.2. The first focus group consisted of local community residents currently between the ages 60 and 75—people regarded as potential future residents. The second group consisted of current ECCRC residents, all of whom were over the age of 80. The responses from the two groups provide valuable insight into what ECCRC is like now and what future residents of ECCRC would like to have.

Community Focus Group (ages 60–75)

Question	Top/Common Answer
Do you know about, and how did you hear about, the CCRC?	From neighbors.
Have you visited this CCRC?	Yes.
Was it your decision to look at this CCRC?	Yes.
Do you think this CCRC meets or will meet your long-term needs?	Not sure. Can't I have these services at home?
Do you think your stay at this CCRC will be temporary?	Yes, I will only need these services for a short time.
Did all the programs and open space at this CCRC make it attractive?	Not sure. Can't I have these services at home?
Did your family encourage you to come to this CCRC?	No, they want me at my home or my daughter's home.
Did you come with your spouse?	Not for the first visit, because my husband says he is not interested in moving, despite his physical limitations.
Did you financially plan to pay for your fees at this CCRC?	Yes.

Current Residents Focus Group (ages 80+)

Question	Top/Common Answer
Do you know about, and how did you hear about, the CCRC?	From discharge folks at the hospital.
Had you visited this CCRC before you moved in?	Yes.
Was it your decision to look at this CCRC?	Not at first. It was my daughter who came with me to visit.
Do you think this CCRC meets or will meet your long-term needs?	Yes.
Do you think your stay at this CCRC will be temporary?	No, this is my home for life.
Did all the programs and open space at this CCRC make it attractive?	Yes.
Did your family encourage you to come to this CCRC?	Yes.

EXHIBIT 13.2
Findings from ECCRC Focus Groups

(continued)

EXHIBIT 13.2
Findings from
ECCRC Focus
Groups
(continued)

Question	Top/Common Answer
Did you come with your spouse?	Yes, but he was very sick and only stayed a year before he died.
Did you financially plan to pay for your fees at this CCRC?	I hope I have enough.
What was the primary reason you are considering or considered this CCRC?	After I visited, I realized I could not stay at home alone.

Strategic Plan

The board has requested that the strategic plan include analyses of five factors affecting the organization's future: (1) population, (2) financing, (3) workforce, (4) healthcare systems, and (5) innovation. Scenarios are to be developed for the two time frames specified.

Your consulting firm has been provided with the focus group and demographic data that ECCRC had already compiled. The consultants will need to incorporate information from additional resources (such as those listed at the end of this case) into their scenarios. The board wants to know that the plan will be "state of the art," so rigorous citations and documentation of evidence-based results, rather than vague or ambiguous statements, are requested. The executive committee of ECCRC has detailed the scope of the work for the consulting contact, which will require answers to the following questions across the five factors.

1. Population
Exhibit 13.1 contains relevant demographic data for this part of the analysis.

    a. For the targeted geographic area in this community, what is the percentage of residents in the following two age groups?
        i. People aged 80 or older
        ii. Members of the baby boomer generation
    b. Does each target population still want an ECCRC-type product?
    c. Is the wealth of this community sufficient and/or improving to be able to pay for a traditional CCRC model of service?
    d. Is the population stagnant, or is the population projected to change significantly because of migration into or out of the community?

2. Financing

    a. How will each of the two age groups pay for long-term care services (i.e., will the current methods we use for healthcare services be available for each of these groups)? What could happen if a reduction of Medicare and Medicaid services occurs?

b. Will Medicare, Medicaid, and Social Security still be available in 2046? Will the Medicare Trust Fund run out of money? What is the forecast for the nation's Social Security budget?

c. What payment arrangements are desired by future target audiences for the CCRC style of living? What income level will a person or couple need to afford each payment model?

d. Should private insurance be incorporated into the payment structure? Will opportunities to be paid by Medicare and Medicaid require that ECCRC obtain various licenses? If so, what are the financial costs of meeting the licensing requirements?

3. Workforce

Most direct caregivers in current long-term care organizations (roughly 80 to 90 percent) are unlicensed but certified nurses' aides. The other nursing positions are filled by licensed staff, including registered nurses and practical nurses, who are allowed by law to pass medications. The majority of other employees—such as maintenance workers, dietary staff, laundry staff, and groundskeepers—are unlicensed semiskilled workers. Turnover for these unlicensed workers is high, as both pay and perceived community respect are low, and the work can be physically and emotionally demanding.

The county has 32 high schools. None are vocational technical high schools, but three have health tracks with practical nursing education. The high school population is about 125,000, with 55 percent minority students. A county-level community college has five campuses, one of which is dedicated to healthcare. That campus has a large nursing program that prepares students to take the state exam to qualify as a registered nurse.

Given that background, the questions to be answered are the following:

a. Will there be sufficient numbers of the various types of workers for each of the two time frames?

b. What is the pipeline (i.e., the current training plans and programs) for future workers? In the past, many skilled and semiskilled workers in long-term care have been immigrants. But if immigration is more difficult and US unemployment levels are low, where will these workers come from?

c. Should ECCRC develop a relationship with the school system for internships or summer jobs to help its employee pipeline?

The US Department of Labor and the National Association of Workforce Boards provide useful resources relevant to these issues, and the American Hospital Association, LeadingAge, and the American Health Care Association all have written extensively on these topics. The board expects these sources to be referenced in the strategic plan, as an indication that national trends have been considered.

4. Healthcare Systems

Every day, the number of mergers and acquisitions of healthcare providers grows, and the number of freestanding healthcare organizations becomes smaller. Many free-standing hospitals of the past are now part of networks or systems. A similar trend is occurring in post-acute care, where more and more single-owner facilities are merging with other facilities.

    a. What is the Aging Network? In addition to healthcare services, what other services might be included?

    b. Should CCRCs merge with other healthcare providers? If so, should the merger be horizontal (i.e., a merger with similar facilities in other areas of the region or country) or vertical (i.e., a merger with a hospital or other healthcare provider entities in the CCRC's own community)?

    c. What are the implications for ECCRC of the growth in innovative payment models for bundled healthcare and support services, such as accountable care organizations?

    d. Should ECCRC consider partnering with an insurance company that offers long-term care insurance?

The American Hospital Association, LeadingAge, and American Health Care Association provide valuable information about these topics. The Centers for Medicare & Medicaid Services and the US Government Accountability Office also have reports that comment on the restructuring of the healthcare field and its impact on services for seniors. The chair of the ECCRC Finance Committee has read the reports and expects that the strategic plan will reflect the issues raised by these nationally recognized entities.

5. Services and Innovations

The board would like the consultants to use the principles of marketing—particularly those pertaining to product life cycle, new products, and entrepreneurship—to examine the potential for innovations in service delivery by ECCRC. Specifically, consultants should consider the following areas:

    a. Lifestyle expectations, with activities revamped to appeal to healthy, active seniors (activities to attract "younger seniors" may include golf outings, pickle ball, on-site gym access, and performing arts initiatives)

    b. Technology-friendly facilities in which seniors of all ages, as well as staff, have high-speed internet service and wi-fi throughout all indoor and outdoor areas

    c. Application of new technologies, such as telemedicine, robots, and smart home technology for the physical plant

    d. Expansion of home and community-based services, including clinical, home care, and homemaker services

e. Access to new treatment modalities and services, including those for dementia and Alzheimer's disease

f. End-of-life care, including hospice and palliative care

Conclusion and Recommendations

The board would like the consulting group to incorporate all of these issues, along with any other salient facts or trends, into a SWOT analysis (i.e., an analysis of strengths, weaknesses, opportunities, and threats) that clearly and concisely depicts ECCRC's challenges and opportunities. The board would also like the full strategic plan, with all of its details and appendices, to include a succinct executive summary. Finally, the board would like the consultants to provide explicit recommendations about what actions ECCRC should take to position itself for success in both the first and second time frames.

Questions

Fact and Data Analysis Questions

1. What is strategic planning?
2. What is marketing? What are the "four Ps" of marketing? How is advertising different from marketing? Use the four Ps to explain what a CCRC is.
3. What is product life cycle? Why is it relevant to this case?
4. Who is the target audience (or target audiences) for this case?
5. Are the demographic data in exhibit 13.1 sufficient for the strategic plan? If not, what other data should be presented to the board? What data are available from secondary sources? What information might be worth the expense of primary data collection?
6. Prepare a table, based on current data, that demonstrates what the payment mix will be for each of the two time frames requested by the board.
7. What is a SWOT analysis? How can it help the board make decisions about the future direction of ECCRC?
8. Define *long-term care.*
9. What are ADLs and IADLs?
10. What are the components of a community's long-term care system? How does a continuum of care differ from long-term care?
11. What subpopulations require long-term care? Do all these subpopulations use the same services?

Discussion Questions

1. If a board amasses data that show convincingly that the products an organization produces are no longer in demand, what are its options regarding the future of the organization?
2. Is long-term care for seniors provided more effectively if seniors reside in their community or if they reside in a CCRC or other institution? Consider efficiency versus quality. How are these issues affected by location?
3. Apply the continuum of care model to a CCRC. How does the conceptual model inform the elements that ECCRC must offer in the future?
4. Contrast quality of life with quality of care.
5. What will be the future for the CCRC model of care for seniors?

Useful Resources

- Administration on Aging (www.aoa.gov)
- American Fact Finder (www.americanfactfinder.gov)
- American Health Case Association (www.ahcancal.org)
- American Hospital Association (www.aha.org)
- Kaiser Family Foundation (www.kff.org)
- LeadingAge (www.leadingage.org)
- US Census Bureau (www.census.gov)

RURAL HEALTHCARE ACCESS AND PHYSICIAN RECRUITMENT

Donald Lewis

Case at a Glance

Overarching theme	The overarching theme of this case is the application of human resource principles for the recruitment and retention of healthcare professionals in rural areas.
Learning objectives	• Contrast the demographic, economic, environmental, and health status characteristics of rural communities and urban communities. • Compare the healthcare systems of rural communities with those of urban communities. • Outline the essential components of human resource management and how these functions are carried out in small organizations. • Analyze the characteristics of and the needs for various disciplines within the healthcare workforce. • Articulate the issues related to recruitment of physicians and other healthcare providers to rural areas. • Develop a workforce recruitment program for a rural area.
Key terms	• Critical access hospital (CAH) • Health Professional Shortage Area (HPSA) • Human resources • Medically Underserved Area (MUA) • Mission • Nonmetropolitan • Rural • Safety net hospital • Stark Law • Telehealth • Vision

Management competencies	Human resources, health workforce analysis, health systems analysis
Population/subgroup	Residents of rural communities
Health issue or condition	Access to healthcare services

Management Challenge

The County Council for Wyoming County was in a state of despair. The latest physician who had been assigned to the county by the National Health Service Corps (NHSC) had just announced that he had completed his commitment and would be leaving in three months. The CEO of Wyoming County General Hospital, Nate Wellworth, had just presented the situation to the council as an emergency addendum to the otherwise routine meeting agenda.

With this physician's departure, Dr. Sara Ramirez, the wife of a local rancher, would now be the only remaining doctor serving the county and its critical access hospital (CAH). Luckily, the council members knew that Dr. Ramirez would be a permanent member of the community, because her family would never give up their ranch. However, she had emphasized that she was an obstetrics and gynecology specialist and did *not* want to be called out in the middle of the night to tend to rattlesnake bites or gunshot accidents. The council implored the hospital CEO to do something to ensure the viability of the CAH and give the local residents access to medical care.

As the senior administrator of a small healthcare organization in a rural[1] area, Nate played many roles. He now had to assume the functions that a director of human resources would conduct in a larger organization. Nate had to come up with a plan to recruit more physicians—full-time, part-time itinerant, telehealth—any means would do!

Background

The provision of high-quality, cost-effective healthcare services depends on the availability of clinically trained personnel. The workforce needed to effectively maintain a population's health includes the following roles:

- Physicians—all specialties
- Operating room technicians
- Nurses (registered nurses and licensed practical nurses)
- Nursing assistants
- Advance practice nurses
- Physician assistants

- Nurse anesthetists
- Medical technicians
- Laboratory technicians
- Radiology technicians
- Paramedics and emergency medical technicians
- Pharmacists
- Physical therapists
- Occupational therapists
- Home health aides
- Respiratory therapists
- Dentists
- Dental hygienists
- Speech therapists
- Public health and health promotion experts
- Social workers

The problem in Wyoming County focused specifically on the availability of physicians. However, many of the challenges associated with recruiting and retaining physicians in rural areas apply for other health personnel as well. Next time, the crisis could be for more nurses, or for a dentist. Nate, the hospital CEO, knew he could not manage Wyoming County's problem alone. He simply did not have the resources to bring on a new physician—let alone find someone in less than three months—or continue to recruit the entire spectrum of health professionals single-handedly.

Nate explained that the reason he brought this issue to the County Council was because the issue affected everyone in the community. The members of the council included the head of a local bank, the principal of the high school, a housewife, a retired Army colonel, and the wife of the local newspaper's editor. Nate recommended convening an emergency task force to muster the creativity and persuasion of as many community factions as possible. Perhaps the appropriate response to the current crisis was not simply adding one more doctor, but rather creating a new vision of health and healthcare in Wyoming County.

At this point in time, Wyoming County General Hospital did not employ physicians directly. However, the urgent need for a primary care specialist caused Nate to rethink the physician staffing model. The hospital might need to offer employment to physicians if it hoped to attract and retain them in sufficient numbers. (Hospital employment of physicians is legal in Wyoming, unlike in some other states.) Nate was also considering the hiring of midlevel practitioners, such as physician assistants or certified nurse practitioners, to help meet the community's primary care needs. Physicians from a major health system had been providing specialty services to the community on an itinerant basis, in space leased from the hospital. Perhaps their services could be increased, if the financial incentives could be structured in a more positive way.

The County Council authorized Nate to prepare a brief plan detailing who should be on the task force and what will need to be done to save the community's access to primary care. Nate decided he would start by educating the task force about human resources (HR) as a management function, what laws are involved, how HR is conducted in a small organization, and why the community and its culture are important (Riedel 2004). The physician recruitment process would need to begin immediately, so convening and educating the task force quickly was imperative.

Aware that the hospital was a driver of the local economy, Nate felt that educating the council about the local multiplier effect of money spent by the hospital would help make the case for a robust recruitment effort (Truit 2004). In general, every dollar the hospital spent locally on wages/salaries, equipment, and other goods and services would have a threefold impact on the local economy. The hospital's expense budget was $40 million per year. Therefore, the local economic impact was $120 million.

To assist the task force with its deliberations, Nate first charged his staff with finding data on (1) how many health practitioners of various specialties are practicing in Wyoming County and (2) what ideal practitioner–population ratios would be. Nate did not want to overburden his staff, but he knew he had to present a comprehensive plan to the County Council that would bring about sustainability of the health workforce, not just a solution for the immediate problem. He had heard at an American College of Healthcare Executives meeting that telehealth offered potential to augment the availability of services in rural communities, so he added the development of a telehealth plan to the agenda. (The terms *telehealth* and *telemedicine* are often used interchangeably.)

Examples of Organizations That Need to Recruit and Retain Physicians in Rural Communities

- Hospitals
- Community mental health centers
- Hospice services
- Rural health clinics
- Veterans Administration clinics
- Indian Health Service units
- Community health centers
- Federally Qualified Health Centers
- Skilled nursing facilities
- School-based clinics
- Home health agencies
- Prison facilities

Although Nate had worked at the Wyoming County General Hospital in various capacities for 14 years, he had only been CEO for two. He had never studied health workforce ratios. It's about time, he thought. Wyoming County needs to know how dire its condition is!

Nate also knew the importance of assessing community assets. Any potential physician recruit, as well as the County Council itself, would want to know what healthcare-related organizations existed in the local area and what additional demands beyond routine clinical care a new doctor should expect. Moreover, Nate thought that the county might have resources that could contribute to primary care but had been overlooked or underutilized.

The State of Rural Healthcare

Nate had assembled some information that he intended to use to educate the County Council about rural healthcare in general:

- According to the US Department of Agriculture (USDA 2013), the United States had 1,976 rural counties and 1,167 metropolitan counties in 2013.
- More than 51 million Americans live in areas classified by the US Office of Management and Budget (OMB) as "nonmetropolitan" (USDA 2012). They make up one-fifth of the US population.
- Residents 65 or older make up about 15 percent of the rural population—a significantly higher percentage than in the urban population (Bailey 2012).
- Rural health disparities have been linked to geographic isolation, lower socioeconomic status, higher rates of health-risk behaviors, and limited job opportunities. Rates of chronic illness and poor overall health are higher in rural communities than in urban populations (Rural Health Information Hub 2019).
- Less than 11 percent of the nation's physicians practice in rural areas. More than 20 million US residents live in areas that have too few physicians to meet their basic needs for healthcare (Federal Office of Rural Health Policy 2019).
- In nonmetropolitan areas, 54 percent of physicians are in the primary care specialties of family or general practice, general internal medicine, pediatrics, and obstetrics/gynecology. In metropolitan areas, only 38 percent of physicians are in those specialties (Federal Office of Rural Health Policy 2019).
- Between 2013 and 2017, 64 rural hospitals closed—more than twice the number from the previous five-year period (US Government Accountability Office 2018).
- "Frontier counties" have been defined as those with a population of fewer than 7 people per square mile, and they account for nearly half of the land mass of the United States (Rural Health Information Hub 2018).

- About 640 counties—roughly 20 percent of the nation's residential areas—are without quick access to an acute care hospital (Williams 2013).
- Nearly 82 percent of rural counties are classified as Medically Underserved Areas (MUAs), which include Health Professional Shortage Areas (HPSAs). According to the Health Resources and Services Administration (HRSA 2019b), as of July 2019, the United States had 6,433 primary care, 4,602 mental health, and 5,320 dental HPSAs.
- According to the American Hospital Association (2019), Medicare and Medicaid accounted for 56 percent of rural hospitals' net revenue in 2017, and this percentage can be extrapolated to other rural providers. Physicians practicing in rural areas will typically see more Medicare and Medicaid beneficiaries than their urban counterparts. Physicians affiliated with rural or urban safety net hospitals will see more Medicaid patients on average (America's Essential Hospitals 2019).

Nate had just become a member of the National Rural Health Association (NRHA) and found the following statement on their website: "Economic factors, cultural and social differences, educational shortcomings, lack of recognition by legislators and the sheer isolation of living in remote areas all conspire to create health care disparities and impede rural Americans in their struggle to lead normal, healthy lives" (NRHA 2019).

Personal Perspective

Jim and Maude Perkins, ages 69 and 67, had lived their entire lives in rural Wyoming County. They married when Jim was 20 and Maude 18, and they had four children, all of whom left the area upon completing high school. Jim ran a successful farm supply business until he retired three years ago.

Jim and Maude had enjoyed relatively good health until the past few years. Jim now was struggling with congestive heart failure and severe arthritis. Maude was having difficulty hearing, and her vision—always poor—had gotten worse with cataracts. They had Medicare and a supplemental health plan, and they had selected a $0 premium Medicare Advantage Plan to minimize monthly costs.

The only trouble was that, to access any service provider, they needed a referral from the primary care physician they had selected when they signed up for the Medicare Advantage Plan. Maude and Jim were both patients of the physician who was leaving the area. Now they are worried about how their medical needs are going to be met.

Human Resources and Recruitment

Management of human resources is arguably the single most important management function of any healthcare organization. In a typical hospital, 70 percent of the budget goes to paying people—nurses, physicians, housekeepers, dietary personnel, security, and a long list of healthcare professionals of various disciplines. Despite advanced technology and expensive equipment, healthcare is a business of service. If providers are not available, not satisfied with their jobs, not organized efficiently, or not compensated adequately, service suffers, quality declines, and patients report negative experiences.

Healthcare organizations, no matter how small or large, must manage HR so that they attract a workforce adequate in skills and capacity, create a positive work environment, and comply with the myriad laws and regulations governing employees and employment. The functions of HR include job analysis, recruitment, retention, training, performance assessment, reward assignment, succession planning, and support for a positive work environment (Riedel 2004).

Recruitment, in particular, is central to the challenge facing rural areas.

Recruitment to Rural Areas

Rural communities vary significantly in size and scope, and rural healthcare organizations need to understand their service/market areas from a healthcare needs perspective, as well as from a lifestyle perspective.

When an organization recruits a physician, it is competing in a national market, with a wide variety of organizations seeking to attract the best available talent. The recruitment effort should be all about selling the opportunity and the lifestyle to potential candidates. The organization may also, in effect, have to recruit the candidate's family or significant other. Many recruitment efforts have failed when family needs were not taken into consideration from the outset.

Recruiting physicians is expensive. Whether done in-house or outsourced, or a combination of the two, recruiting a single physician can easily cost upward of $20,000 to $50,000 dollars, once all expenses and fees are taken into consideration. Healthcare organizations—particularly those in rural areas—cannot afford to throw away that money by recruiting with a lack of due diligence on the front end of the process. Recruitment expenses are not covered by Medicare.

The Recruitment Process

Establishing a recruitment process that is proactive and well thought out goes a long way to help ensure success. Some rural facilities that are big enough to have their own in-house recruiting departments do all of their own sourcing and coordination of visits. Most rural facilities, however, do not have full recruiting departments. Instead, they have staff who are responsible for overseeing the recruiting process and, more often than not, contract with recruiting agencies to source candidates.

Potential Issues in Rural Communities That Affect Recruitment of Physicians and Other Health Professionals

- Small size and remote geographic location
- Physician shortages and scarce workforce
- Acute lack of access and availability of care
- Lack of transportation, public or private
- High percentage of elderly and poor residents
- Limited access to capital for state-of-the-art equipment
- Limited availability of high-tech infrastructure and services
- Regulations, both federal and state
- Reimbursement issues
- Lack of high-quality schools
- Employment opportunities for spouse or significant other
- Possible push-back from existing physicians
- Lifestyle considerations

If the organization chooses to retain a recruiting agency, the agency first must be vetted. The organization should seek to establish a working relationship with a recruiter who understands the organization, the community, and the realities of rural healthcare. Recruiting agencies work on either a contingency basis, in which the agency represents the physician, or a retained search basis, in which the agency represents the organization. The type of approach selected will affect the time, effort, and support received from the firm. It also determines the costs.

Process Steps for Wyoming County to Consider

The Wyoming County task force delineated the steps for an effective recruitment process. By making a list, the task force could assign responsibilities, be transparent about what resources the community needed to provide, determine a time frame, and spread the recruitment process among community members beyond just the CEO and C-suite staff of the hospital.

The list included the following:

- Establish a recruitment committee made up of key stakeholders as appropriate (e.g., administration, medical staff, the board of directors). Wyoming County could use the County Council or the task force for this purpose, or it could create an entirely new committee. The task force pondered which members of the community should be formally recognized in the process, and which should be involved in informal ways.
- Create a vision statement for the recruitment program.

- Produce a recruitment video that could be distributed via DVD, flash drive, and the internet. Aware that producing a professional-looking video would take expertise and good equipment, the task force thought it might be able to work with the state bureau of tourism or attract contributions from the public (e.g., through a local contest for "best photography"). The local school kids, as well as retirees and tourists, always seemed to find great pictures to share.

- Make sure the organization's website and other relevant websites are up to date. In a rural area where "everyone knows everyone," keeping up a website is often not viewed as a high priority—except during tourist season. However, an accurate online presence would be important to the recruitment process. The task force made a list of all the sites that would need to be current, and it considered engaging the local high school to make the website improvements into a project, with a pizza party as the reward.

- Determine physician workforce needs based on a medical staff needs analysis, the age of existing physicians, planned retirements, outward migration for care, discussions with physicians who serve the residents of Wyoming County, and a community health needs assessment. This assessment should include all the immediately adjacent counties, as well as those on the interstate highway to the nearest large city.

- Determine practice style (e.g., solo, group practice, employed, fee-for-service) and practice location.

- Establish recruitment parameters with regard to income guarantees, salary, sign-on bonuses, medical school loan repayment, relocation expense, working capital loans, management services organization (i.e., practice management support), and marketing. Features to attract physicians must comply with all Internal Revenue Service and Stark Law regulations.

- Determine sourcing approach—in-house, contingency (representing the physicians), or retained (representing the organization)—and offer a bonus to current physicians and employees for successful leads.

- Select a realtor to do community and housing tours. Educate realtors about the importance of the physician recruitment process to the community's well-being.

- Work with local schools to be part of the recruitment site visit.

Telehealth and Rural Healthcare

Nate had put "telehealth" on the initial list that he presented to the County Council. The initial reaction was, "What's this? Why is it relevant?" Nate responded with the following points:

- People coming out of medical school today are much more interested than their predecessors were in maintaining a work–life balance.

- No one can be on call 24 hours a day, 7 days a week.
- Often, a rural area has only one physician in a given specialty.
- The lack of colleagues in a specialty area can be an impediment to recruiting.
- Patient volume in a given service area might not be sufficient for a physician to maintain a high skill level and/or make a living.
- Access to continuing medical education can be difficult due to time and distance parameters.

Telehealth offers the potential to address these and other concerns, improving patients' access to services while balancing physician workload, minimizing isolation, and providing access to continuing education online.

Patient Success Stories Related to Telehealth

- A 33-year-old woman presented to the emergency department (ED) of a rural Wyoming hospital with classic stroke symptoms. The hospital did not have a neurologist on staff, but it did have a telestroke program with an urban medical center. Through use of the program, the patient was able to receive the appropriate medication. Instead of dying or becoming disabled from a stroke, the woman went home to her family.
- A rural South Carolina hospital was located several hours from the nearest urban area, and no psychiatric service providers were nearby. When patients would arrive in the ED in a psychiatric crisis, they would be seen and put in a holding room. On average, a psychiatric consult could not be done until seven to ten days later. After the hospital started a telepsych program with an urban hospital, the wait time was reduced to a matter of minutes.

The major medical center that was providing specialty care coverage in the Wyoming County community on an itinerant basis also had a robust telehealth program. However, unlike other rural hospitals in the state, Wyoming County General Hospital had never considered using that service to meet the community's primary or specialty care needs. Nate knew that the use of telehealth warranted serious consideration.

The availability of telehealth can alleviate many of the concerns that have made recruiting for rural healthcare difficult. Colleagues and consultants from anywhere in the world can be available 24/7, which can mitigate rural practitioners' sense of isolation. Patient visits, follow-up, and many specialist services can be done via telehealth, which can help minimize coverage concerns for local medical staff.

The Office for the Advancement of Telehealth (OAT), within the HRSA, provides grants for telehealth equipment. The OAT program has four rural health objectives (HRSA 2019a):

1. Improving access to needed services
2. Reducing rural practitioner isolation
3. Improving health system productivity and efficiency
4. Improving patient outcomes

Federally funded Telehealth Resource Centers throughout the United States help rural organizations and providers implement cost-effective telehealth initiatives. Rural organizations that need to create a telehealth program but lack the broadband infrastructure to do so can contact the Universal Service Administrative Company (USAC) Rural Healthcare Program, which contributes funding for the development of rural healthcare broadband infrastructure (USAC 2019). The US Department of Agriculture also provides grant funding for telehealth equipment.

Conclusion

The recruitment of physicians and other health professionals to rural areas is a challenge. However, every practice opportunity and rural community has unique benefits to offer to health professionals, whether they are new graduates or experienced practitioners. Rural communities are wonderful places to raise a family. Crime tends to be lower, people look out for one another, outdoor activities are numerous, and the overall quality of life is good. The right match between a healthcare provider and a community is out there, and Wyoming County needs to commit to making it happen.

Questions

Fact and Data Analysis Questions

1. What are the primary functions of a human resources department?
2. What percentage of physicians practice in rural communities?
3. What is a HPSA, and how much does Medicare increase a physician's payment for practicing in a HPSA?
4. What is the NHSC?
5. What is the Stark Law?
6. Where is the health-provider-per-population ratio found for each health professional discipline? On what basis are ideal provider–population ratios established?

7. What data sets offer information pertaining to the distribution and availability of health professionals? (Provide names, data, and website addresses.)

Discussion Questions

1. How does human resource management in healthcare organizations differ from HR management in other types of industries?
2. What can be done to mitigate the challenges associated with recruitment of physicians to rural areas?
3. How is recruitment of other types of health professionals the same as or different from recruitment of physicians to rural areas?
4. Why is it so important to have access to at least one physician in a rural area? If no physician is available, what substitutes exist?
5. What steps would you take to create a physician recruitment program? What will be the succession planning component of the program?
6. What stakeholders would you include on a physician recruitment committee for a rural hospital, and why?
7. How can the community become involved in the recruitment of physicians?
8. How would you determine the benefits that telehealth might contribute to a recruitment program?
9. How can social media be leveraged to enhance a physician recruitment program?
10. What elements are most important to worker satisfaction? How can these elements be incorporated into an HR plan for a healthcare organization in a rural area?
11. What are five key pieces of legislation that govern employment in the United States, and how do they apply to the healthcare industry?
12. How do obligations differ for physicians who are employed by a hospital and physicians who have privileges to work at a hospital but are not employed by it?
13. What can healthcare organizations do to retain physicians and staff, once recruited?
14. Conduct mock interviews for the recruitment of a health professional to practice in a rural area. What questions would you ask specific to the rural area? What criteria would you use to rate candidates?

Note

1. A variety of definitions of the word *rural* are used by the federal government and/or researchers. Throughout this case, the terms *nonmetropolitan* and *rural* are used interchangeably.

References

American Hospital Association (AHA). 2019. *Rural Report: Challenges Facing Rural Communities and the Roadmap to Ensure Local Access to High-Quality, Affordable Care.* Published February. www.aha.org/system/files/2019-02/rural-report-2019.pdf.

America's Essential Hospitals. 2019. "Essential Data: Our Hospitals, Our Patients." Published April 11. https://essentialhospitals.org/institute/essential-data-our-hospitals-our-patients/.

Bailey, J. 2012. "Medicaid and Rural America." Center for Rural Affairs. Published February. http://files.cfra.org/pdf/Medicaid.pdf.

Federal Office of Rural Health Policy. 2019. "Facts About Rural Physicians." Cecil G. Sheps Center for Health Services Research, University of North Carolina at Chapel Hill. Accessed July 11. www.shepscenter.unc.edu/rural/pubs/finding_brief/phy.html.

Health Resources and Services Administration (HRSA). 2019a. "Agency Information Collection Activities: Submission to OMB for Review and Approval; Public Comment Request; Information Collection Request Title: Telehealth Resource Center Performance Measurement Tool, OMB No. 0915-0361-Revision." Published February 5. www.federalregister.gov/documents/2019/02/05/2019-01107/agency-information-collection-activities-submission-to-omb-for-review-and-approval-public-comment.

———. 2019b. "Shortage Areas." Accessed July 11. https://data.hrsa.gov/topics/health-workforce/shortage-areas.

National Rural Health Association (NRHA). 2019. "About Rural Health Care." Accessed July 11. www.ruralhealthweb.org/about-nrha/about-rural-health-care.

Riedel, J. 2004. "Human Resources." In *Managing Long-Term Care,* edited by C. Evashwick and J. Riedel, 43–69. Chicago: Health Administration Press.

Rural Health Information Hub. 2019. "Rural Health Disparities." Reviewed April 22. www.ruralhealthinfo.org/topics/rural-health-disparities.

———. 2018. "Health and Healthcare in Frontier Areas." Reviewed June 7. www.ruralhealthinfo.org/topics/frontier.

Truit, T. 2004. "Why the 'Local Multiplier Effect' Always Counts." Grassroots Economic Organizing. Accessed July 10, 2019. www.geo.coop/archives/LocalMultiplierEffect1104.htm.

Universal Service Administrative Company (USAC). 2019. "Welcome to the Rural Health Care Program." Accessed July 11. www.usac.org/rhc/.

US Department of Agriculture (USDA). 2013. "Rural-Urban Continuum Codes." Published May. www.ers.usda.gov/data-products/rural-urban-continuum-codes/documentation.aspx.

———. 2012. "Gap in Population Growth Rates for Rural and Urban Areas Continues to Widen." Updated September 11. www.ers.usda.gov/data-products/chart-gallery/gallery/chart-detail/?chartId=76050.

US Government Accountability Office. 2018. "Rural Hospital Closures: Number and Characteristics of Affected Hospitals and Contributing Factors." Published August 29. www.gao.gov/products/GAO-18-634.

Williams, J. P. 2013. "What Happens When a Town's Only Hospital Shuts Down?" *U.S. News & World Report.* Published November 8. https://health.usnews.com/health-news/hospital-of-tomorrow/articles/2013/11/08/what-happens-when-the-only-hospital-closes.

Useful Resources

- American Hospital Association—Fact Sheet: The Economic Contribution of Hospitals (www.aha.org/2010-06-17-fact-sheet-economic-contribution-hospitals)
- American Hospital Association—Small and Rural (www.aha.org/taxonomy/term/147)
- Centers for Medicare & Medicaid Services—Community Mental Health Center (www.cms.gov/Research-Statistics-Data-and-Systems/Downloadable-Public-Use-Files/Cost-Reports/CMHC-.html)
- HealthIT.gov—Resources for Critical Access Hospitals and Small Rural Hospitals (www.healthit.gov/topic/health-it-health-care-settings/resources-critical-access-hospitals-and-small-rural-hospitals)
- Health Resources and Services Administration—Federal Office of Rural Health Policy (www.hrsa.gov/rural-health/index.html)
- Health Resources and Services Administration—Telehealth Programs (www.hrsa.gov/rural-health/telehealth/index.html)
- Indian Health Service (www.ihs.gov)
- *The Journal of Rural Health* (https://onlinelibrary.wiley.com/journal/17480361)
- Kaiser Family Foundation—State Health Facts (www.kff.org/statedata/)
- National AHEC Organization (www.nationalahec.org)
- National Association of Counties (www.naco.org)
- National Consortium of Telehealth Resource Centers (www.telehealthresourcecenter.org)
- National Health Service Corps (https://nhsc.hrsa.gov)
- National Organization of Sate Offices of Rural Health (https://nosorh.org/)
- National Rural Health Association (www.ruralhealthweb.org)
- "Physicians and Rural America," by Roger A. Rosenblatt and L. Gary Hart, *Western Journal of Medicine*, November 2000 (www.ncbi.nlm.nih.gov/pmc/articles/PMC1071163/)
- US Department of Agriculture Economic Research Service—Rural Classifications (www.ers.usda.gov/topics/rural-economy-population/rural-classifications.aspx)
- US Government Accountability Office—Rural Hospital Closures (www.gao.gov/products/GAO-18-634)

COMMUNICATION AND MARKETING: LIVE WELL SAN DIEGO

Wilma J. Wooten, Elizabeth Evashwick, Nick Macchione, Carleen Stoskopf, and Dale Fleming

Case at a Glance

Overarching theme	This case focuses on how a healthcare organization can apply the principles of marketing and communication to reach individuals, partner organizations, leaders, and other stakeholders.
Learning objectives	• Prioritize target audiences. • Create messages appropriate for an identified audience. • Select media effective for messages and target audiences. • Manage the process of encoding and decoding messages. • Apply metrics for measuring media and message effectiveness. • Monitor communications for cultural sensitivity and health literacy. • Develop a communications plan for a health program.
Key terms	• Communication process • Cultural competence • Decoding • Encoding • Health literacy • Marketing • Noise • Social marketing • Social media • Target market/audience
Management competencies	Communications, marketing
Population/subgroup	San Diego County citizens
Health issue or condition	Varied

Management Challenge

Sarah is a newly hired director of marketing and communications for Balboa County, and her charge is to develop a communications plan that reaches all of the stakeholders of county programs—in particular, the community and its residents. Sarah knows a lot about marketing and communications in general, but she is new to public health. She is looking for exemplary communication plans by health organizations and for examples of effective communication strategies that incorporate data into messaging. If she is going to request funds for the next annual budget cycle, she must submit a preliminary plan to her boss, the director of the public health department, within the next three months.

Background

During the course of her research, Sarah has found the website for Live Well San Diego (www.livewellsd.org), a San Diego County program that emphasizes a regional vision for communities that are "Building Better Health, Living Safely, and Thriving" (Live Well San Diego 2019a). Live Well San Diego employs a model based on the vital

As Easy as 3-4-50

San Diego County's health and human services director, Nick Macchione, wanted to find a way to address the underlying conditions that play such an important role in a community's health. He wondered why San Diego, like so many places, was spending so much on healthcare and not seeing results. What was contributing to poor health in the community? And how could the county and its community partners address the problem? As a result of asking these questions, Live Well San Diego as a project was born.

Macchione and his team adopted the 3-4-50 principle, which became the foundation for Live Well San Diego's Building Better Health component. This principle states that three behaviors (poor diets, physical inactivity, and smoking) contribute to four chronic diseases (cancer, heart disease and stroke, diabetes, and respiratory conditions) that contribute to more than 50 percent of deaths. Based on this concept, the team directed the county to focus on encouraging three simple behaviors that can have a major impact: healthy eating, exercising, and stopping smoking.

The 3-4-50 principle proved useful for promoting healthy choices, fostering policy and environmental change, and persuading community leaders and organizational partners to join with Live Well San Diego. For more information on the 3-4-50 principle, see Waters (2013).

principles of cross-sector partnerships, collective impact, and community engagement. The common element across all these principles is communication. Sarah is considering whether Balboa County could benefit from creating a similar model. She has learned that social marketing differs from business marketing in its goals and approaches, and she wonders if a model such as Live Well San Diego's can be successful for both.

The San Diego County Board of Supervisors adopted Live Well San Diego in 2010. At that point, it was a proposed ten-year plan to advance the health, safety, and well-being of the region's more than 3 million residents. Today, Live Well San Diego is a regional vision owned by partners across various sectors of government, schools, businesses, media, and community and faith-based organizations.

Live Well San Diego consists of three components: Building Better Health, adopted on July 13, 2010; Living Safely, adopted on October 9, 2012; and Thriving, adopted on October 21, 2014. Having begun with only with the health component, county leadership soon realized that the program needed to expand to focus on building a sense of safety and achieving a good quality of life.

Live Well San Diego measures its success through ten main indicators stratified across five areas of influence. The first area of influence is Health, which includes two indicators: life expectancy and quality of life. The second area is Knowledge, which includes an education indicator. The third area, Standard of Living, includes indicators for unemployment rate and income. The fourth area, Community, has three indicators: security, physical environment, and built environment. Finally, the fifth area, Social, includes indicators for vulnerable populations and community involvement (Live Well San Diego 2019c). These and other indicators serve to measure the county's collective efforts to promote well-being across the life span.

The structure of Live Well San Diego is based on recognition that no single agency, on its own, can improve the health of a population in an area as large and diverse as San Diego County. The program's leaders understood the importance of reaching out to communities throughout the region and engaging them to identify and adopt community health improvement plans that would achieve results.

The development of partnerships has been critical to the success of Live Well San Diego. In 2018, Live Well San Diego had 429 named partner organizations. The partners include cities and tribal governments; diverse businesses, including those in healthcare and technology; military and veterans organizations; schools; and community and faith-based organizations. The organizations participate by measuring, documenting, and tracking the results of the policies and programs they implement. The ten indicators are monitored annually to determine the degree of change occurring in the community over time.

The Live Well San Diego model engages its partner organizations as influencers, who may in turn reach out to constituents, members, or residents of the county. Partners and stakeholders from across the various sectors encourage San Diegans of all ages to stay active, eat well, not smoke, take care of their mental health, and get connected to quality care when needed. Efforts in each of these areas have had a positive impact on the Live Well San Diego health indicators.

For example, analysis of the impact of various activities, in 2017, showed the following:

- 4,100 San Diegans were reached via Facebook for mental health focus groups.
- 200 parents learned how to make nutritious and affordable meals.
- 23,000 high school students were trained to recognize signs of depression and suicide.
- 1,000 students viewed presentations on dental health.

A prominent feature of Live Well San Diego (2019b) is its website and data portal. Exhibit 15.1 shows a section of the website that tracks the two indicators for the Health area of influence—life expectancy and quality of life—across various San Diego neighborhoods. Exhibit 15.2 shows the dashboard on which the ten indicators are displayed.

EXHIBIT 15.1
Live Well San Diego Indicators Across Various Neighborhoods

Top 10 *Live Well San Diego* Indicators

The Top 10 *Live Well San Diego* Indicators define what it means to live well in San Diego. Measured across the lifespan among all residents, these Indicators capture the collective impact of programs, services, and interventions using evidence-based practices to create a region where all residents are healthy, safe and thriving. The table below represents the progress being made by all partners across the North County Regions.

			Indicator Performance				Trend is moving in the right direction ↑↓				Trend is moving in the wrong direction ↑↓							
Indicator	Trend	San Diego County	North Coastal Region - (NCR)	North Inland Region - (NIR)	Carlsbad - NCR	Oceanside - NCR	Pendleton - NCR	San Dieguito - NCR	Vista - NCR	Anza-Borrego Springs - NIR	Escondido - NIR	Fallbrook - NIR	North San Diego - NIR	Palomar-Julian - NIR	Pauma - NIR	Poway - NIR	Ramona - NIR	San Marcos - NIR	Valley Center - NIR
HEALTH																		
Life Expectancy: Average life expectancy for a baby born today (2016)	↑	82.1	83.3	82.7	83.7	81.9	U	85.6	82.2	U	81.0	81.5	85.2	U	73.4	83.5	82.8	82.4	82.5
Quality of Life: Percent (%) of people healthy enough to live independently (2016)	↑	94.8%	95.3%	94.8%	95.6%	94.2%	99.5%	96.1%	95.5%	85.0%	94.4%	93.2%	95.9%	93.1%	95.5%	95.7%	95.5%	94.4%	95.3%

Source: Used with permission from Live Well San Diego.

EXHIBIT 15.2
Live Well San Diego Dashboard

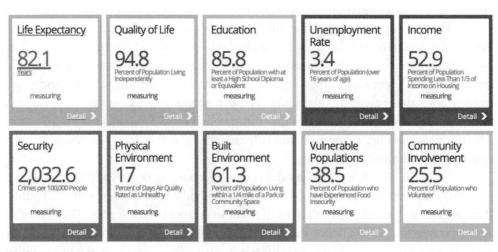

Top Ten Indicators

Life Expectancy
82.1
Years
measuring
Detail >

Quality of Life
94.8
Percent of Population Living Independently
measuring
Detail >

Education
85.8
Percent of Population with at least a High School Diploma or Equivalent
measuring
Detail >

Unemployment Rate
3.4
Percent of Population (over 16 years of age)
measuring
Detail >

Income
52.9
Percent of Population Spending Less Than 1/3 of Income on Housing
measuring
Detail >

Security
2,032.6
Crimes per 100,000 People
measuring
Detail >

Physical Environment
17
Percent of Days Air Quality Rated as Unhealthy
measuring
Detail >

Built Environment
61.3
Percent of Population Living within a 1/4 mile of a Park or Community Space
measuring
Detail >

Vulnerable Populations
38.5
Percent of Population who have Experienced Food Insecurity
measuring
Detail >

Community Involvement
25.5
Percent of Population who Volunteer
measuring
Detail >

Source: Used with permission from Live Well San Diego.

Sarah is impressed with the amount of data that Live Well San Diego has aggregated, but she questions whether that type of model would meet the communication needs of Balboa County. She is charged with reaching out to the residents of her county, and she has assumed that the effort will require sending messages to people directly. Sarah must admit, however, that the Live Well San Diego approach—of engaging community leaders and partner organizations to develop health messages designed for their specific constituents—seems like an effective way of maximizing resources to reach the greatest number of people with messages that are meaningful to them.

The Communication Process

As she approaches her task, Sarah considers the basics of the communication process, modeled in exhibit 15.3. The process begins with Sarah as the marketing director. She is the source, or sender, of the message through which Balboa County will communicate with the community.

Sarah first must *encode* the message—in other words, she must transform the county's abstract ideas and goals into a communicable message that will resonate with the intended target audience. Given what she knows about her community, she wants to use a combination of worded messages and graphics to appeal to people of all levels of education and speakers of different languages. She is aware that

EXHIBIT 15.3
Communication
Process

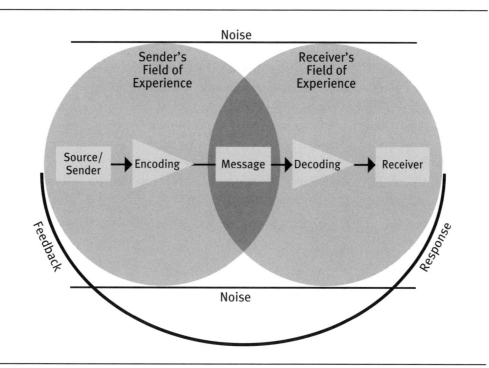

the degree of health literacy varies among Balboa County's residents. The audience will hopefully receive the message and *decode* it, understanding its intended meaning. Sarah is considering using a website as the channel of communication for the message.

In the case of Live Well San Diego, residents who visited the program's website would ideally come to an understanding that the county is promoting community health and has resources to help its residents get and stay healthy. The Live Well San Diego website does not, however, have information about specific diseases and health conditions. That level of information is available through other online sources, such as the federal Centers for Disease Control and Prevention and commercial websites such as WebMD.

Sarah hopes to receive feedback from her target audience once the website has been created. Feedback can take the form of either communication or behavior in response to the message. Sarah will need to be able to measure feedback if her website is to be a useful marketing tool. She hopes to make the website clear and easy to use. Anything that disrupts the communication or prevents the audience from receiving or understanding the message is considered *noise* and should be avoided.

Keys to Effective Communication

Sarah, as a marketing and communications director, knows that the keys to effective communication are to have a comprehensive communications plan and to emphasize transparency. Targeting her message to specific audiences will be important, because the same message may need to be crafted differently for different groups, or even translated into different languages, to reflect cultural competence.

Initially, Sarah thinks that she may need two different messages. One message would be aimed at the stakeholders of county programs, and it would focus on the impact the programs are having on the community. The other message would address Balboa County residents and seek to inform them directly about programs available in the county. Her plan will need to be adaptable to allow for feedback and improvement.

Sarah follows a communication process centered on the following five questions:

- Who is the target audience?
- What is the message?
    - Information
    - Education
    - Question
    - Call to action

- Are the encoded and decoded messages the same? (For example, is language translation appropriate?)
- What potential distractions (i.e., noise) in the environment could hinder communication?
- Did the message get received and interpreted correctly?

With regard to the first question, Sarah knows her target audiences well: They are the stakeholders of county health programs and the residents of Balboa County. Understanding these groups' characteristics and the ways they think will be crucial for effective communication. Sarah believes the people she is trying to reach are ready for change and will be receptive to a message about community health.

Sarah's data on Balboa County indicate that about 80 percent of the residents speak English and 20 percent list Korean as their primary language. The county also has a large senior population. Data show that 50 percent of Balboa County residents will first look to the internet for their healthcare concerns. Given these characteristics, Sarah knows any website the county creates will need to have a user-friendly interface and multilingual tools.

Live Well San Diego has dealt with similar audience concerns, given San Diego County's multilingual population and large number of senior residents. The program has created bilingual informational bulletins and handouts, as well as a Viva Bien San Diego brand for non-English speakers. Live Well San Diego reaches out to the senior population through its Age Well action plan, which seeks to create age-friendly, dementia-friendly communities by changing policies, systems, and environments.

Live Well San Diego reaches stakeholders by embedding its logo in public posters, publications, and informational videos, as well as through media partnerships that point people to the website. Public events (e.g., blood pressure checks, five-kilometer runs/walks, community-based depression screenings) also help draw visitors to the website for registration, health education, and event locations, with the goal of encouraging them to explore other areas of the website as well. Special campaigns, such as 31-day challenges, encourage the public to sign up for emails with clickable health reminders that take participants directly to the website. In addition, social media platforms such as Facebook can be used to advertise the website to particular geographic locations and demographics at a relatively low cost.

With regard to her message, Sarah wants to market the programs that Balboa County offers while also tracking their impact on the community. Live Well San Diego has a similar mission, although its focus expands beyond healthcare to include overall health and wellness. Live Well San Diego maintains a public-facing county website that provides program information to residents through an array of mechanisms. The data portal enables both individuals and organizations to track progress on the ten top indicators and to observe the impact from policies, systems, and environmental changes over time.

Live Well San Diego's portal both *harnesses* and *humanizes* data to improve outcomes. Harnessing data involves gathering data in a way that respects the privacy of residents and customers, while also making that data available in a way that makes sense for members of the community, regardless of their interests or professions. Humanizing data involves fostering a greater understanding of the humans behind the data, along with the priorities, policies, resources, and actions that will positively affect them.

Live Well San Diego shares its harnessed data through blogs, newsletters, Facebook Live, LiveStories, and other strategies, as well as through face-to-face meetings of the leadership teams working to develop, implement, and track their community health improvement plans.

Choosing Metrics

Live Well San Diego applied a set of guiding principles and followed a painstaking process for the selection of the ten health indicators it would track. County leaders wanted indicators that were reliable and reproducible; measurable at federal, state, local, and subregional levels; and collected on a regular basis. Sarah, however, is new to healthcare communications and uncertain of what metrics would be most important in evaluating the effectiveness of her communications plan. She does not yet know what the best practice is.

Sarah is considering whether to (1) measure the effectiveness of a particular type of media (e.g., how many hits a website gets) or (2) look at measures of the health status of the community. She is aware that pursuing the second option—and collecting sufficient data to see any patterns that flow from her marketing plan—would require a long-term, sustained intervention. Alternatively, she is also considering a third approach—somewhat in between the other two—that could involve measuring short-term reactions. For example, after a period of promoting and marketing immunizations, she could track the immunization data to look for a subsequent net increase.

Which of these three options would give Sarah the best and most useful data in terms of reflecting the community's health and the efficacy of the county's healthcare marketing? Which method should she choose?

Choosing Media

Sarah recognizes the importance of matching the media to the target audience. In considering the media through which to communicate her message, she thinks of the Live Well San Diego data portal, which has the most recent demographic, economic, behavioral, and health data (e.g., communicable diseases, noncommunicable diseases, injuries, maternal and child health) for the various communities in San Diego County. Sarah finds the idea of a data portal interesting, but she questions whether the residents of Balboa County would know what to do with this data, or whether they would understand how the data apply to them. Healthcare stakeholders would likely find this resource useful, but they are a more sophisticated audience; Sarah wants to reach lay individuals in her county.

Sarah is thinking the major part of her budget will go toward electronic media. However, the county's older Korean population is an important demographic for her to reach, and many older Koreans do not speak English or use computers as much as other adults. Sarah thinks the Korean newspaper in town might offer an alternative method of communicating with this group, so she is considering allocating some of her budget and energy toward creating ads and articles for this newspaper, as well as other media outlets. If she does, she faces another decision: Should the ads and articles themselves offer health information, or should they just direct people to the website? Sarah has a limited budget and wants every marketing communication to have as great an impact as possible.

Social Media Marketing

A hospital believes that its clients search for recommendations and healthcare providers on social media, so it asks Noah, the hospital's marketing director, to create social media accounts to better reach the community. Noah's goal is to use social media to engage clients, expand awareness of the hospital's programs, and improve the credibility of the hospital.

Live Well San Diego also uses social media accounts to promote its message, and it has had success with various social media campaigns across numerous county departments and programs. One initiative in particular that has effectively engaged the county and community partners via social media is "Love Your Heart Day," an annual blood pressure screening program. More than 200 partners participate to conduct screenings for employees, patrons, clients and patients.

What tactics should Noah incorporate into his social media marketing to promote the hospital, and why? What are the downsides of using social media in marketing?

Media Budget

Crafting the media budget is another critical step for Sarah as she plans her communications. When making the budget, she must use an evidence-based approach to media selection and know the costs of the tools she wants to use.

Given the appropriate budget, a website similar to the one used by Live Well San Diego could certainly be practical. However, Sarah would need to ensure that a "Live Well Balboa" site would be accessible for Balboa County's various community members. It would need to be simple and easy to navigate, have adjustable font size, and offer varying languages. Working with her county offices for communications and information technology, Sarah could determine the costs of replicating the San Diego project on a scale appropriate for Balboa County.

Conclusion

Sarah is impressed with the information and resources that Live Well San Diego provides its community, the way the program has created a network of partner organizations and engaged communities, and the way that it tracks the community's health. Nonetheless, she is still uncertain whether creating a similar resource for Balboa County would produce the results the county health department has specified in its community health improvement plan for the coming year.

Questions

Fact and Data Analysis Questions

1. What stakeholders (i.e., target audiences) should be included in a health organization's communications plan?
2. What data can be used to identify the optimum media for reaching a given target audience?
3. What are the four main types of messages that health or public health organizations might send?
4. What does it mean to "encode" and "decode" a message?
5. How does cultural competency apply to communications?
6. What is health literacy? How does it relate to the messages that Sarah might craft?
7. Give examples of metrics for measuring use of media.
8. Compare the prices of using various types of media to reach the same target audience. How would you determine which method was the most cost-effective?

Discussion Questions

1. What are the differences between marketing to a "community" and marketing to a defined population subgroup?
2. What are the strengths and weaknesses of Live Well San Diego's approach to communicating the importance of healthy behaviors to residents throughout the community?
3. What elements should be included in a communications plan?
4. What would happen if various organizational partners of Live Well San Diego took different approaches to healthy behaviors and sent out conflicting messages? Would anyone have the authority to arbitrate the messages? Who would determine the "correct" message?

5. Consider the ten indicators used by Live Well San Diego. Do the indicators tell you everything you would want to know about the health of the population? Would they all change at the same rate and in the same direction, if the goal is to trend changes over time? What other measures might a county want to track about residents' health status?

References

Live Well San Diego. 2019a. "About Live Well San Diego." Accessed July 16. www.livewellsd.org/content/livewell/home/about.html.

———. 2019b. "Data & Results." Accessed July 16. www.livewellsd.org/content/livewell/home/data-results.html.

———. 2019c. "Top Ten Live Well San Diego Indicators." Accessed July 16. www.livewellsd.org/content/livewell/home/data-results/Indicator-Home.html.

Waters, R. 2013. "It's as Easy as 3-4-50: San Diego Works to Change Its Culture, Improve Its Health—and Live Well." *Forbes.* Published December 4. www.forbes.com/sites/robwaters/2013/12/04/its-as-easy-as-3-4-50-san-diego-works-to-change-its-culture-improve-its-health-and-live-well/.

Useful Resources

- Centers for Disease Control and Prevention—Gateway to Health Communication and Social Marketing Practice (www.cdc.gov/healthcommunication/index.html)
- Centers for Disease Control and Prevention—Health Literacy (www.cdc.gov/healthliteracy/index.html)
- Live Well San Diego (www.livewellsd.org)
- *Marketing Health Services* (Health Administration Press, 2014), by Richard K. Thomas

16

STRUCTURE AND GOVERNANCE FOR SUSTAINABILITY: MANAGING RESURGENCE OF HIV/AIDS IN A COMMUNITY

Keith Jennings

Case at a Glance

Overarching theme	The focus of this case is on how to structure a multi-entity program for long-term sustainability.
Learning objectives	• Identify ways of organizing community health resources to address health problems that cross institutions.
	• Analyze interentity structural and process factors affecting the sustainability of community health programs over time.
	• Articulate the terms of an interentity agreement between health provider organizations.
	• Explain how clinical advances can affect the diagnosis, treatment, and prevention of a given health condition.
	• Analyze how trends in health conditions affect the organization of a community's health system.
	• Evaluate methods of care coordination and case management.
	• Analyze the business case for a health organization to be involved with its community.
Key terms	• Care coordination
	• Managerial epidemiology
	• Memorandum of understanding (MOU)
	• Ryan White Act
	• Sustainability
	• SMART objectives
Management competency	Organizational behavior
Population/subgroup	People with HIV/AIDS
Health issue or condition	HIV/AIDS

Management Challenge

Dale Jones is the CEO of Whitefield Health System (WHS); Susan Hernandez is the director of the local public health department (LHD) for the region; and Shay Zodpey is the head of the Positive Response Initiative (PRI), a local organization committed to fighting HIV/AIDS. The three are meeting for coffee to discuss how to approach a new problem—the sudden reemergence of HIV in their community.

Community institutions had worked together in the preceding decades—before Jones, Hernandez, and Zodpey had started in their management roles—to control HIV and to manage people living with HIV or AIDS. The three leaders now agree that they need to reinvigorate the community collaboration of the past and develop an infrastructure that can sustain community efforts to prevent and manage HIV/AIDS into the future.

Background

Today, two trends are fueling a resurgence of HIV/AIDS in communities throughout the United States. The first is a rise in injection drug use (IDU). The second is the arrival of a younger generation that is less likely to get tested for HIV (Howard 2018). If the past is an indication of the future, health system and other community health leaders must proactively evaluate the ever-changing scientific and cultural shifts surrounding HIV/AIDS and strategically adapt their collective response accordingly.

Chronic, complex conditions such as HIV/AIDS require collaboration across multiple health and social service agencies. Jones, Hernandez, and Zodpey, therefore, recognize that addressing the HIV/AIDS resurgence will require a community effort and an adaptive approach. The art of structuring and managing collaborative relationships is an essential management competency, though it often goes unrecognized. Developing such relationships requires skill as well as resources (e.g., staff time, the cost of patient services that might not be billable to third-party payers, communication expenses, political capital). Moreover, the relationships need to be nurtured over time and altered as needed when external and internal conditions (especially leadership) change. The three leaders will have to continually evaluate HIV/AIDS's changing landscape and respond in sustainable ways to drive measurable impact.

Managerial epidemiology—the science of managing health services based on the changing health conditions of a community—has become increasingly important for health and social service organizations, and it will be essential for addressing the resurgence of HIV/AIDS. Healthcare executives need to closely monitor community health status to tailor their services to individuals and the community, maximize the use of resources, and improve financial performance.

The History and Epidemiology of HIV/AIDS

Managing HIV/AIDS from an institutional perspective requires an understanding of the history of the condition and the efforts to diagnose, treat, and prevent it. Because HIV is an infectious condition that morphs into a complex chronic condition, a dual approach to prevention and management is essential.

HIV—which stands for *human immunodeficiency virus*—is a virus that attacks the body's immune system via the CD4 cells, also known as T cells (Centers for Disease Control and Prevention 2019). The virus spreads through certain bodily fluids and, over time, can destroy enough cells that the body can no longer rebound and heal, allowing other infections or cancers to take advantage of the body's weakened state. If left untreated, HIV can lead to acquired immunodeficiency syndrome, or AIDS.

During the 1980s, AIDS made headlines and spurred hysteria throughout the United States. Specific groups soon became stigmatized, particularly those in what came to be known as the "four-H club": homosexuals, heroin users, Haitians, and hemophiliacs (Nall 2018). Patients often were abandoned by their families and left to healthcare entities and charity organizations. Given the lack of available treatment options at the time, the primary objective of the local healthcare community was to help the people dying from AIDS to have as much dignity as possible in their death. Hospitals and newly formed hospices provided the vast majority of care unilaterally to people with AIDS (Nall 2018).

The 1990s brought incredible leaps in awareness, education, funding, and treatment breakthroughs related to HIV and AIDS. The focus of the local healthcare community shifted from providing dignity in death to helping patients manage the difficult side effects of drug therapies. This dramatic shift brought a new set of challenges to local communities, including how to treat, house, feed, transport, employ, and insure a growing group of people in crisis, while also reducing the spread of infection. Community agencies that had previously not worked together suddenly became allies in caring for people with multifaceted needs. The Ryan White Comprehensive AIDS Resources Emergency (CARE) Act, enacted by the federal government in 1990, provided various categories of government funding (Health Resources and Services Administration 2019), but it offered no guidance about coordination. Case management approaches developed over time through both formal and informal arrangements.

HIV/AIDS epidemiology is continually evolving. Despite significant progress in decreasing the overall impact of the disease, certain populations—such as racial and ethnic minorities and low-income rural areas—carry a greater share of the burden. Three subgroups that face a particularly high risk of HIV/AIDS are substance users (especially users of hard drugs); men who have sex with men (sometimes called the MSM population); and recent immigrants, particularly from Latin America.

Another key aspect of managing HIV/AIDS is care coordination, or case management. *Care coordination* refers to assistance provided to individuals to help them access the various clinical and support services they need. The care coordination role has emerged over the past several decades to become a formally recognized position—one that select payers will now pay for. Information systems to facilitate coordination of care and to document services provided by multiple organizations and professionals remain scarce, but they are increasingly regarded as essential for the efficient provision of care and success in value-based payment.

Systems for managing HIV/AIDS require that health and social services, managerial epidemiology, and care coordination be pulled together. The challenge facing Jones, Hernandez, and Zodpey is how to create cross-entity partnerships that will incorporate these elements and enable the community to effectively battle HIV/AIDS on an ongoing basis.

HIV/AIDS Reemergence

A staff member in the local public health department responsible for maintaining the infectious disease registry had become concerned that the number of HIV cases in Whitefield's three-county region was increasing. The region historically sees 150–200 new cases per year, which averages to about 15 new cases each month. However, according to a review of the data, the past three months had seen 27, 32, and 41 newly diagnosed HIV patients, respectively. Similar surges in confirmed HIV cases were being reported in other surrounding regions. Soon, state health officials and the Centers for Disease Control and Prevention (CDC) became involved.

After investigating patient records, the epidemiologists of the public health department determined that injection drug use was the root cause of about 80 percent of the new HIV cases. All the patients who reported IDU identified oxymorphone as their drug of choice, though some reported injecting methamphetamine and heroin, as well. Coinfection with hepatitis C was diagnosed in 85 percent of the IDU-associated cases.

Public health nurses and staff from agencies affiliated with the Positive Response Initiative questioned patients about partners who might have been exposed through syringe sharing, sexual encounters, or other high-risk activities, and local public health teams tried to locate and test any individuals named. About two-thirds of those potentially exposed individuals were located and tested; about one-third declined or were unable to be tested.

Another key factor in controlling the HIV upsurge was the implementation of a needle exchange program (also known as *syringe access*). Providers caring for people with HIV discovered that IDU practices centered around crushing and cooking 40-milligram oxymorphone tablets and then injecting. Drug preparation equipment and insulin syringes were frequently shared, with the number of injection partners being as high as six per injection event.

Behaviors associated with IDU have instigated a new HIV epidemic in communities around the United States, challenging the historic structures of many community programs focused on HIV/AIDS prevention and treatment. Managing HIV/AIDS in a community comes at a significant cost. Illinois, a state severely affected by new IDU-driven HIV diagnoses, reported that, if no action is taken, the cost of providing lifetime care for the projected infections between 2018 and 2030 would amount to $6.7 billion, with much of the burden falling on Medicaid (AIDS Foundation of Chicago 2018).

A Cluster of Infections

A population facing high levels of IDU-driven HIV infection has more to worry about than HIV itself. HIV is a cluster of infections coupled with coinfections and other challenges. Hepatitis B and C, skin disease associated with needle reuse, overdose deaths, and various other issues require significant resource infrastructure from the local healthcare community. According to the CDC, tuberculosis is the leading cause of death for people with HIV/AIDS, accounting for 40 percent of deaths among people living with HIV in 2016 (CDC Division of Global HIV and TB 2018).

In 2017, the CDC identified 52 clusters of HIV transmission (Office of HIV/AIDS and Infectious Disease Policy 2017). Many recent outbreaks of HIV have occurred in rural populations that have had a historically low risk of HIV infection (Rudavsky 2016). The virus has spread quickly through IDU within highly networked groups, putting a unique burden on local health systems.

In the wake of the renewed HIV/AIDS threat, teams participating in local prevention and treatment efforts must find new ways to manage the spread of HIV, while also improving the quality of life for people infected and at risk. At the same time, community health leaders and partners must evaluate whether their respective investments through funding, staffing, and other resource contributions are creating enough value to justify continued investment. Furthermore, they must determine what moral and ethical roles they play in serving populations that bear a disproportionate share of the burden of HIV's spread.

Jones, Zodpey, and Hernandez realize now that their community has grown complacent about HIV/AIDS. Young people are no longer being bombarded with messages about cautionary behavior and testing, and even older members of the community have largely moved on from the AIDS scare of the past. The community needs to wake up!

Community Overview

The Whitefield Health System, the local health department, and the Positive Response Initiative provide services for a three-county region in the southeastern United States. The area is predominantly rural with two suburban pockets, with a total population of 211,500. Median household income ranges from a high of $57,300 in the largest county to $39,400 in the smallest. Less than 15 percent of residents have a college degree.

Poverty is pervasive in the region. Empty storefronts and strip malls litter the highways and town squares. Area mills that had employed community members for generations have eliminated many low-skilled jobs, often replacing them with automation.

The primary mode of HIV transmission in the region has been men having sex with men (61.5 percent of cases), followed by heterosexual contact (27.1 percent) and IDU (7.5 percent). Patients are most often male, and newly diagnosed patients are most often under the age of 30. However, like many areas of the country, the region is facing a significant increase in IDU. It has also experienced a recent influx of immigrants, particularly from Mexico and South American countries, exacerbating the HIV/AIDS problem.

Did You Know?

- More than one in four people who inject drugs reuse needles (Boerner 2018).
- Some families have three generations of users shooting up alongside one another.
- In winter, as many as 10 to 20 users have been known to live in a single dwelling that has heat. In summer, the same can happen in a dwelling that has air-conditioning.
- Sharing needles is common practice; people often reuse needles until they break.
- Addiction can be so powerful that the sensation of a needle prick can bring relief.

About Whitefield Health System

Whitefield Health System has a 250-bed inpatient facility and three clinics in outlying rural areas. With 2,200 employees, it is one of the larger employers in the region. The affiliated physician medical group has a wide range of specialists, but it does not have extensive depth. Primary care and emergency physicians are in demand at WHS, as they are throughout the nation.

Care for patients with HIV/AIDS is an important responsibility for the health system but also a financial burden. These patients typically consume considerable resources, often are uninsured, and frequently fall into the hospital's community benefit contribution for uncompensated care. Reducing the burden of HIV/AIDS in the community is of great interest to WHS, both for the sake of people's well-being and for its own bottom line. However, one challenge with making HIV/AIDS a priority is that the community health needs assessment (CHNA) and WHS's own patient records show that the region's top healthcare problems are heart conditions, cancer, stroke, and dementia.

Dale Jones, the CEO, has been with WHS for more than 35 years, since the early days of the initial HIV/AIDS outbreak, and he has seen the community response evolve over time. But up until five years ago, he was a practicing clinician, not an administrator.

The Local Public Health Department

The local public health department serves two of the three counties in the region, including those where the greatest outbreak is occurring. (For historic reasons, the state's economic planning regions do not line up with the state public health regions.)

The majority of state public health efforts are spearheaded by government agencies and the state university, based in the state capital—which is 200 miles away from the region served by this LHD. The state does not maintain an extensive budget for public health. In terms of visibility, power, and public health funding, the area of the state served by this LHD typically plays second fiddle to other areas. The LHD has assumed responsibility for leading the CHNA for the two counties it covers, as required by the Public Health Accreditation Board for LHD accreditation. This effort also satisfies the hospital's requirement to complete a CHNA every three years to qualify for tax-exempt status.

Susan Hernandez, the LHD director, received her doctorate in epidemiology from the state university's school of public health. She is new to the director role, having served previously in surveillance.

Positive Response Initiative

The Positive Response Initiative began in the 1980s, when a group of volunteers came together to form "care teams" to support people in the community who were dying from HIV/AIDS. PRI was formed as a collaboration between WHS and the local Public Health Nursing Association (PHNA), and it received initial funding from the state health department.

PRI continues as a stand-alone entity with tax-exempt status. Its board of governors includes representatives from WHS, the LHD, the PHNA, and four other community agencies. PRI's CEO is a nurse, Shay Zodpey, who had served in a clinical capacity providing patient care until the previous CEO retired. Zodpey's exposure to management is strictly limited to his work with patient care teams.

From its inception, PRI has had three primary objectives: (1) to offer patients dignity and self-determination, (2) to connect them with care options, and (3) to provide the highest quality of life possible. Throughout the past 30 years—even as treatment breakthroughs and cultural shifts have rendered many other HIV/AIDS service organizations ineffective or obsolete—PRI has remained committed to these three objectives, while also evolving its programming, operations, and funding to remain relevant.

From a structural perspective, PRI is a portfolio of five service lines of programs and funding—(1) prevention, (2) basic needs, (3) medical needs, (4) support groups, and (5) giving back—bound together by a mission to provide preventive and prescriptive HIV services. It serves the HIV-positive population and populations at high risk for HIV infection (e.g., the MSM population, people with substance abuse issues, the local Latino community). Services targeted at high-risk subgroups cross-cut the five service lines.

Personal Perspective

Steven is a new resident of the Whitefield community. A young man with a history of substance abuse, he had recently relapsed and was attending a 12-step meeting at the local Life Recovery Center (LRC), one of the Whitefield Health System's community partners.

On the day of the meeting, the hospital's prevention team was on-site at LRC providing education and testing, and Steven decided to sit in and listen. After hearing about the risk behaviors associated with HIV, he made the decision to learn his status. The center performed a rapid HIV test (a preferred method for people with substance use disorder, who may be difficult to locate days later), and the Positive Response Initiative's health educator completed Steven's risk assessment. Twenty minutes later, a staff member informed Steven that his result was preliminary positive.

While completing a blood draw to confirm the test results, the team spoke with Steven about PRI's services and the importance of having a support system. The team learned that Steven was currently homeless and living in his car after being terminated from his drug treatment program following a relapse. The team provided Steven with a gas voucher to cover his transportation expenses and asked him to come to PRI's office the following day to check in.

Once Steven was confirmed to be HIV-positive, his care coordinator began linking him with PRI's core service areas, starting with housing. A bed was reserved for him at a local homeless shelter until one of PRI's subsidized housing units became available.

(continued)

Steven was assigned to a substance abuse counselor who employs a harm reduction approach to treatment, without the threat of termination. Under the safety of this approach, Steven was honest about his drug use and began working on a recovery plan. Within a few months, he was placed in subsidized housing and provided with a meal delivery program, offered in partnership with a local food pantry.

Once Steven's basic needs had been met, the PRI team was able to address the medical issues associated with his HIV infection. His care coordinator helped him apply for a state medical program and connect with a local infectious disease physician. He began antiretroviral therapy (ART), which involved a difficult adjustment to the side effects of medication. His care coordinator provided ongoing support throughout the treatment program.

Steven joined one of PRI's local support groups for HIV positive individuals, and he attended many of its social and educational sessions. In time, once he felt ready, he was able to secure a part-time job. He eventually served as a member of PRI's speakers bureau and spoke at a local awareness event on World AIDS Day.

Stories similar to Steven's occur in communities throughout the United States each day. What is critical for health system and public health leaders to understand is that the discovery of HIV in community members is not the primary objective when managing a resurgence. Discovery is just the first step. The real focus is helping at-risk community members live longer, healthier lives through creative, sustainable community partnerships.

Service Lines

Each of PRI's five core service lines is critical in responding to the HIV/AIDS resurgence and managing patients' journey to long-term health and quality of life. None of the service lines is offered by PRI alone; all require PRI to coordinate with other organizations in the community. WHS is one of PRI's key partners.

Prevention

PRI teams, which are actively present at partner locations in the region, provide education and testing, with the goals of increasing public knowledge of HIV risk reduction, ensuring early disease identification, and decreasing risk behaviors among high-risk individuals who have tested negative.

Basic Needs

Housing, food, transportation, translation/communication, and insurance are essential elements in ensuring that newly diagnosed HIV patients can and will follow through with their treatment plan. Through contractual community partnerships, PRI works to make sure patients have the ability to maintain their treatment regimen.

Medical Needs

Ideally, patients should have access to medications, side-effects management, and individual and group therapy. PRI collaborates with area physicians, therapists, pharmacists, clinics, dentists, and other care teams to ensure continuity of care. As new clinical advances occur relevant to HIV/AIDS, all involved must be educated about the impact of those advances on the prevention, diagnosis, and treatment of the condition, and processes and procedures must be changed accordingly. Constant communication among all parties is essential.

Support Groups

Social and education sessions for people who are HIV-positive create a support system that incentivizes care compliance, helps prevent relapse, restores family relationships, and provides a foundation for employment. PRI offers programming that assists patients with job interviewing and transportation to and from jobs.

Giving Back

Successful patients are the best advocates for HIV prevention in the community. They can also be the best supporters for newly diagnosed patients.

PRI also supports patients and the community through local partnerships with infectious disease physicians, nutritional support services, translation services, low-income housing providers, immigration counselors, and support groups. The goal of an effective HIV/AIDS program is not to "own" the expertise in every area associated with HIV; it is to recognize that HIV-positive patients' needs are as unique as each individual and that successful outcomes require the program to serve each patient through an appropriate network of experts and services.

Funding and Internal Operations

PRI's services are designed under two care coordination teams—Prevention Services and Patient Services—which are active across Whitefield's three-county region.

PRI funding comes from a complex mix of sources. Grants, fee-for-service payment, and other revenue aimed at prevention come from the CDC, the Substance Abuse and Mental Health Services Administration, Whitefield Health System, and private foundations. Funding for client services comes from the federal Department of Housing and Urban Development, the state's Department of Health, Whitefield Health System, and private foundations. Federal funds from the Ryan White Act are particularly important.

A key to PRI's effectiveness has been evolving its approach to partnerships within the communities it serves. PRI has more than 50 written, formalized partnerships in the three-county region, as well as dozens of informal partnerships built primarily through staff-to-community personal relationships. Clinicians and case managers initiate and receive numerous referrals each day. A common approach to structuring formal relationships and boundaries between interentity partners is the use of a memorandum of understanding (MOU). This type of agreement between two or more entities serves situations in which collaborating entities either cannot or do not want to enter into a legally enforceable agreement. An MOU between community partners should be clear, concise, and updated over time. PRI uses a combination of formal MOU agreements, a few legal contracts related primarily to funding, and many informal arrangements. The website and staff use the term "partner" generously, with no precise relevancy to management structures.

PRI maintains rigorous evaluation, with metrics divided into three macro segments: HIV prevention, early intervention, and patient health. The initiative tracks both hard and soft metrics across each of these areas. Together, the metrics provide partners with real-time intelligence on the spread of HIV, as well as the effectiveness of PRI programs in improving the quality of life of HIV-positive patients.

High-Risk Populations

Services for high-risk populations are matrixed across the five service lines. Efforts targeted at particular high-risk groups include the following:

- *The substance-use population.* PRI's Prevention Services team works regularly with county jails, state prisons, health clinics for military veterans, substance abuse treatment centers and programs, and homeless shelters. These partnerships provide access to high-risk substance-using individuals who would generally be unlikely to seek out HIV testing. By being present at these partner sites and providing on-site education and testing, PRI is able to stay at the forefront of HIV's spread. PRI staff are also able to respond immediately to positive tests with access to the Patient Services team.

- *The MSM population.* PRI partners with LGBTQ groups to integrate education into fun, community-building events. For example, instead of passing out condoms and providing traditional health education, PRI has joined forces with LGBTQ groups to host a "Jeopardy"-style sexual trivia game hosted by drag performers at a local gay bar. The event provides education in a nontraditional way, while PRI health educators provide testing at a confidential location inside the bar.

- *The Latino population.* PRI faces multiple barriers in providing services to members of the Latino population, especially new immigrants to the community. Such barriers may include language; cultural taboos; institutional distrust; and a history of limited access to health education, testing, or services. Many individuals feel uncomfortable discussing sexual health, and many also fear interacting with large institutions, such as the local health system. To reach this population, PRI has partnered with more than 20 local restaurants to provide "First AIDS Kits" in kitchen areas, which include basic first aid with condoms and safe-sex information in Spanish.

Sustainability

Sustainability refers to the likelihood that a program or approach will continue to function effectively after initial support (e.g., financial support, community enthusiasm, board favor) comes to an end. Community-based HIV prevention and management are based on breadth and depth of collaborative partnerships, both formal and informal, with services throughout the region. Building the relationship from the start requires following the principles of good partnership management.

Workforce experience and expertise can have a significant impact on sustainability. However, Jones, the Whitefield Health System CEO, finds that he is one of the few "old timers" involved in addressing the current crisis. Hernandez and Zodpey are relatively new. Many of their staff, both management and clinical, only began working in the community in the past decade and are unaware of how or why partnerships had evolved; often, staff had difficulty differentiating formal from informal arrangements. Case managers referred cases back and forth, but the MOUs underpinning those referrals were often out of date. Furthermore, many staff members at health and social service organizations throughout the region

Being SMART About HIV/AIDS

An essential ingredient in PRI's approach to evaluating, responding to, and preventing the spread of HIV is the use of SMART objectives—that is, objectives that are specific, measurable, assignable, realistic, and time related. (Note: Other variations of the SMART concept use slightly different terminology—for instance, specific, measurable, attainable, relevant, and time bound.)

Following the SMART framework introduced by George T. Doran (1981), PRI focuses on the following criteria for its programming:

- *Specific*: The program clearly targets an area for improvement.
- *Measurable*: The program has indicators of progress.
- *Assignable*: The program is clear about who does what.
- *Realistic*: The program knows what can be achieved, given available resources.
- *Time related*: The program is clear about when results can be achieved.

This framework has helped PRI to stay on top of emerging cultural and medical trends and adapt its programming to achieve sustainable and measurable impact. PRI's SMART goals for the recent IDU crisis are substantially different from those used during the 1990s.

were oblivious to new requirements for client confidentiality, information systems management, and financing.

Each decade has offered new challenges for the people responding to surges in HIV infection. No two outbreaks have been the same. Plus, changes in treatment, medicine, and funding require programs and community leaders to adapt their structures, processes, and philosophies to each situation and season. Jones, Hernandez, and Zodpey agree that the current outbreak presents an opportunity to revisit all aspects of the partnership arrangements and to implement revisions that will sustain momentum in HIV/AIDS prevention in the long term.

A Plan of Action

By the time Jones, Hernandez, and Zodpev conclude their coffee meeting, they have drafted a plan of action that includes a vision statement, a short list of overarching long-term goals, and key tasks to be accomplished in the short term. The leaders will now share the plan with their respective boards. They have agreed to return in two weeks to implement revisions from the boards and then proceed to the development of a more detailed plan.

They have also agreed on the following underlying assumptions, to serve as guiding principles for their work:

1. HIV/AIDS prevention and treatment must be a community-wide effort.
2. Numerous organizations must be involved as formal partners and commit to achieving specific community-level goals. The principles of identifying and managing partnerships must be properly employed; random arrangements created by informal agreements between staff do not lead to sustainability over time.
3. Leadership is essential. For the Whitefield region, WHS, the LHD, and PRI will be co-champions. Their partnership agreement must be particularly strong.
4. Development of a crisp vision that can be understood and accepted by lay persons as well as professionals is an essential first step.
5. A work plan will be developed using SMART objectives and detailed tasks, responsibilities, time frames, and resources.
6. An evaluation, with process and outcomes measures, will be agreed upon, and responsibility for and attribution of success will be shared by all partners.
7. A multifaceted, multimedia communications plan is an integral part of the service plan.
8. Financing must be incorporated into ongoing operations, not dependent upon external grants or one-time awards.

The three leaders agree to appoint one staff member to spearhead the plan for each organization, and these three appointees will be the team responsible for delineating how other entities and the community will be involved.

Jones, Hernandez, and Zodpey depart knowing that their task will require considerable effort in the short term but, done right, will benefit the entire community over the long term.

You have been appointed as one of the three members of the team. What are your next steps? What will you put in place to share with the board?

Questions

Fact and Data Analysis Questions

1. Define *managerial epidemiology*. How is it used by healthcare institutions?
2. Who maintains disease registries? Who is responsible for reporting? How can the information in these registries be used by a healthcare provider to plan or manage its services?
3. What is the formal definition of a *chronic condition*? What entity created this definition? Differentiate a chronic condition from an infectious disease.
4. PRI performs five types of tasks. What types of professionals are involved with each?
5. What is the difference between an MOU and a formal contract?
6. What are the roles of the state and local public health departments in monitoring infectious diseases? What are their roles for chronic conditions?
7. What conditions are clinicians required to report to public authorities?
8. What metrics can be used to measure the success of a program addressing multiple facets of HIV/AIDS and multiple subpopulations?

Discussion Questions

1. How has the health system response to HIV/AIDS changed over time? Why? What lessons can healthcare executives learn from this evolution?
2. How does an institution select partners, whether formal or informal? What criteria and processes might be used?
3. What should be in the terms of a formal MOU?
4. What organizational elements are critical to the sustainability of a multifaceted program over time? Do these factors differ if the program involves multiple organizations?
5. What are SMART objectives?
6. How are services for people with HIV/AIDS paid for?

7. What are the economics of HIV/AIDS programming for WHS? Does the health system make or lose money by participating in a community-wide effort to reduce HIV/AIDS?

8. What is care coordination? What mechanisms might PRI and WHS use to coordinate the care for a single individual client? How is care coordination related to institutional partnerships, if at all?

9. How, if at all, does addressing HIV/AIDS at a community level vary from addressing the subpopulations most affected? Differentiate messages, interventions, and outcome measures for programming at a community level from those for programming for the subpopulations at high risk of HID/AIDS.

10. If a vaccine for HIV/AIDS is developed and becomes widely available at an affordable price, how will the activities of PRI change?

References

AIDS Foundation of Chicago. 2018. "A Framework to Eliminate HIV in Illinois." Updated June 6. https://gtzillinois.hiv/wp-content/uploads/2018/06/Getting-to-Zero-Fact-Sheet.pdf.

Boerner, H. 2018. "Mapping How the Opioid Epidemic Sparked an HIV Outbreak." *Shots: Health News from NPR*. Published January 2018. www.npr.org/sections/health-shots/2018/01/14/577713525/mapping-how-the-opioid-epidemic-sparked-an-hiv-outbreak.

Centers for Disease Control and Prevention (CDC). 2019. "About HIV/AIDS." Updated April 24. www.cdc.gov/hiv/basics/whatishiv.html.

Centers for Disease Control and Prevention (CDC) Division of Global HIV and TB. 2018. "How the CDC Is Scaling Up TB Prevention for People with HIV." Published March 23. www.one.org/us/2018/03/23/tuberculosis-hiv-aids-cdc-prevention/.

Doran, G. T. 1981. "There's a S.M.A.R.T. Way to Write Management's Goals and Objectives." *Management Review* 70 (11): 35–36.

Health Resources and Services Administration. 2019. "About the Ryan White HIV/AIDS Program." Reviewed February. https://hab.hrsa.gov/about-ryan-white-hivaids-program/about-ryan-white-hivaids-program.

Howard, J. 2018. "Fewer Young Adults Getting HIV Tests, Here's Why." CNN. Published January 25. www.cnn.com/2018/01/25/health/hiv-testing-trends-cdc-study/index.html.

Nall, R. 2018. "The History of HIV and AIDS in the United States." *Healthline*. Reviewed January 29. www.healthline.com/health/hiv-aids/history.

Office of HIV/AIDS and Infectious Disease Policy. 2017. *National HIV/AIDS Strategy for the United States: 2017 Progress Report*. US Department of Health and Human Services. Accessed July 18, 2019. https://files.hiv.gov/s3fs-public/NHAS_Progress_Report_2017.pdf.

Rudavsky, S. 2016. "An Indiana Town Recovering from 190 HIV Cases." *Indianapolis Star*. Published April 8. www.indystar.com/story/news/2016/04/08/year-after-hiv-outbreak-austin-still-community-recovery/82133598/.

Useful Resources

- *And the Band Played On: Politics, People, and the AIDS Epidemic,* 20th-anniversary edition (St. Martin's, 2007), by Randy Shilts
- US Department of Health and Human Services—A Timeline of HIV and AIDS (www. hiv.gov/hiv-basics/overview/history/hiv-and-aids-timeline)

ABOUT THE EDITORS

Connie J. Evashwick, ScD, LFACHE, is an experienced healthcare administrator, author, and educator who thrives at the nexus of management and academia. Dr. Evashwick holds bachelor's and master's degrees from Stanford University and master's and doctoral degrees from the Harvard School of Public Health. She has been credentialed in public health and association management and is a Lifetime Fellow of the American College of Healthcare Executives. Her areas of expertise include the continuum of care, health professions education, hospital community benefit, and international public health. Dr. Evashwick has taught community and population health for healthcare management programs and has authored more than 110 articles and 15 books.

Jason S. Turner, PhD, is associate dean and associate professor at the Rush University College of Health Sciences. Prior to entering academia, Dr. Turner spent a number of years in the healthcare sector as a controller for a large, national healthcare insurer and as an administrator for a hospital chain. He primarily teaches corporate finance, economics, accounting, leadership and strategy, and population health management to graduate students entering the health services field. Dr. Turner is a Fellow with the Academy of Healthcare Management.

ABOUT THE CONTRIBUTORS

Charles L. Angel Jr. is pursuing a master of science in health administration degree at the University of Alabama at Birmingham.

Sheila Baxter is principal of business development (strategic partnerships) at Kaiser Permanente within the Chief Digital Office. In addition, she currently serves as a board member on the Women Health Care Executives of NorCal and as an advisory board member for ConnectWell. Previously, Baxter was the vice president of business development and marketing for Healthy Communities Institute, where she played an instrumental role in growing the business and developing partner relationships aimed at improving population and community health. She completed her master's in public health in health policy and management at the University of California, Berkeley, where she received the Henrik L. Blum Award for Distinguished Social Action. She also holds a certificate in marketing management from Harvard University.

Jenny Belforte is the chief operating officer for Ceres Community Project. Previously, she was vice president of community health solutions for Conduent Healthy Communities Institute. There, she worked with a diverse group of clients representing hospitals, public health agencies, and community coalitions around the country to implement products and services, including community health needs assessments and implementation strategies. She received a BA degree in psychology from the University of California, Berkeley, and an MPH degree in community health sciences from the University of California, Los Angeles.

Sophia Blachman-Biatch manages her own consulting business with health systems, foundations, and start-ups, with a special focus on addressing the economic determinants of health through community engagement and strategic innovation. Previously, she was an account manager with Conduent Healthy Communities Institute. She holds a BA in psychology and global health, with a certificate of integrated marketing communications, from Northwestern University. She completed her MPH at the Harvard T.H. Chan School of Public Health in 2019.

Margaret Bozik, JD, is the director of asset management and special initiatives at the Champlain Housing Trust. She is responsible for overseeing the performance and financial health of the nonprofit's rental portfolio, which includes about 2,000 apartments and several commercial buildings. She is also a co-chair of the Chittenden County Homeless Alliance and serves on the Governor's Council on Homelessness. Previously, Bozik worked in the Community and Economic Development Office for Burlington, Vermont. She has a law degree from the University of Pittsburgh and is a member of the Vermont bar.

Robert E. Burke, PhD, is professor emeritus at George Washington University's Milken Institute School of Public Health. Dr. Burke has had a distinguished career leading health services research focused on quality, finance, administration, and evaluation for aging services in both the public and private sectors. After moving to academia in 2002, Dr. Burke served as professor and chair in the Department of Health Services Management and Leadership, helping to develop the online executive MHA program and conceiving and teaching an innovative course on community and population health. He holds bachelor's and master's degrees from Boston College and a doctorate in philosophy (medical sociology) from the University of Florida.

Rosemary M. Caron, PhD, is a professor in the Department of Health Management and Policy of the College of Health and Human Services at the University of New Hampshire. Her research is on community-based participation in solving complex urban public health problems, population health as a management approach, and the public health workforce. Prior to entering academia, Dr. Caron worked as a practitioner in a variety of public health settings. She holds a doctorate in pharmacology and toxicology from Dartmouth College, a master's degree in public health from Boston University School of Public Health, and a bachelor of arts degree in chemistry from Regis College.

Chris Donnelly is the director of community relations at the Champlain Housing Trust. He directs the trust's external communications, including community and endowment fundraising, grant writing, media and public relations, coalition and advocacy work, marketing of all programs and homes, and all publications. He also oversees community organizing and member relations. His background is in public policy.

Elizabeth Evashwick is a Presidential Fellow and works for the US Department of State. She is a member of the California State Bar and has worked as a consultant for Pepperdine University School of Law. She holds a JD degree from Pepperdine University School of Law and a BA degree in government and law from Lafayette College.

Dale Fleming retired in 2018 from the position of director of the Office of Strategy and Innovation, a division of the San Diego County Health and Human Services Agency. She worked with the County of San Diego for more than 30 years, serving in various capacities. She was heavily involved in the development of Live Well San Diego, a regional collective impact wellness model, and provided executive leadership for Community Action Partnership, which assists economically disadvantaged communities.

Fleming also provided executive oversight to the agency's media relations team and support for special projects.

Marisue Garganta is director of community health integration for Dignity Health St. Joseph's Hospital and Medical Center. She has more than 40 years of experience in healthcare, community health, education, international business, and nonprofit management. Her roles have included executive director, educator, researcher, trainer, public speaker, and leader in the community.

Allyson Hall, PhD, is a professor in the Department of Health Services Administration at the University of Alabama at Birmingham. She is the program director for her department's graduate programs in healthcare quality and safety. Her research focuses on access to healthcare for vulnerable populations, including low-income populations and individuals living with disabilities. Dr. Hall has a PhD in health policy from the Bloomberg School of Public Health at Johns Hopkins University.

Orna Intrator, PhD, is a professor of public health sciences at the University of Rochester Medical Center, an adjunct professor of geriatrics and palliative medicine at the Icahn School of Medicine, and an adjunct professor at the Brown University School of Public Health. She is the director and research health scientist of the national Geriatrics and Extended Care Data Analysis Center of the US Department of Veterans Affairs (VA). Her VA research focuses on infrastructure to enable studies of the access, quality, and costs of frail veterans' use of VA, Medicare, and Medicaid healthcare programs in the community. Dr. Intrator holds a BSc degree in mathematics and computer science from Tel Aviv University and MSc and PhD degrees in applied mathematics from Brown University.

Penrose Jackson retired in 2018 from the University of Vermont Medical Center (UVM MC). She joined the College of Nursing and Health Sciences to establish a nurse practitioner doctoral program for certification in psychiatric, mental health, and medication-assisted treatment care for patients. Previously, she served for 15 years as the UVM MC director of community health improvement. Jackson received her bachelor's degree from the University of Vermont and a certification in community benefit from Saint Louis University. She was awarded the Association for Community Health Improvement's first Leadership Champion / Spirit of the Community award in 2017.

Keith Jennings is vice president of community impact for Jackson Healthcare in Alpharetta, Georgia. He leads the organization's multifaceted social impact strategy, with a special focus on two priorities: access to healthcare and the well-being of young people. With more than 25 years of healthcare experience on both the health system and vendor sides, Jennings specializes in scaling up new services and businesses. Jennings holds a BA in English literature from Florida State University.

Reena Joseph is a doctoral student in the Department of Health Services Administration at the University of Alabama at Birmingham. She holds a master of health administration degree from the University of Missouri in Columbia and previously practiced as a dental surgeon in India.

Andrew Juhnke is the compliance officer and data product manager for the California Health Interview Survey at the University of California, Los Angeles, Center for Health Policy Research. He oversees compliance coordination, data access confidentiality security, data production and dissemination, and research support and coordination. Juhnke has experience with community health needs assessments—specifically, the data collection, analysis, and synthesis components—from his time as a research associate at Conduent Healthy Communities Institute. He holds a BA in political science from Stanford University and an MPH degree with a concentration in global health from Emory University's Rollins School of Public Health.

Bruce Kinosian, MD, is an associate professor of medicine at the Pearlman School of Medicine and an associate of the Leonard Davis Institute of Health Economics of the University of Pennsylvania in Philadelphia. As associate director and research health scientist of the national Geriatrics and Extended Care Data Analysis Center of the US Department of Veterans Affairs (VA), he has developed cost and utilization projection methods calibrated to frail elderly populations and also validated and refined a frailty index (the JEN frailty index) for use in the VA. Kinosian holds a baccalaureate degree in economics from Stanford University and an MD degree from the University of California, San Francisco.

Donald Lewis, LFACHE, is a professor in the master of health administration programs for George Washington University and Champlain College. He has more than 40 years of senior healthcare leadership experience, including 25 years as a CEO for a rural hospital. He holds an MHA from George Washington University and is board-certified in healthcare management.

Claire Lindsay is a senior health planner with the Office of Policy and Planning for the San Francisco Department of Public Health. Previously, she was a public health consultant with Conduent Healthy Communities Institute, with a focus on policy writing and legislative strategic planning, building and facilitating coalitions and collaboratives, and community health research and evaluation. She holds a BS in nutrition from California Polytechnic State University and an MPH in epidemiology and community health sciences from Boston University.

Nick Macchione is the director of the San Diego County's Health and Human Services Agency. He also oversees the operations of the county's psychiatric hospital, the Edgemoor Skilled Nursing Facility, a children's emergency shelter, and a residential high school for foster youth. For more than 20 years, he has been an instructor and faculty member at San Diego State University's Graduate School of Public Health. Macchione has served as a community strategist, convener, and leader of large-scale population-based health improvements—most notably through the ambitious Live Well San Diego initiative. Macchione holds dual master's degrees from Columbia University and New York University, as well as a senior healthcare leadership certificate from Harvard University.

Bernard R. (Bert) Malone retired in 2016 after 41 years of public health service, which included employment at the federal, state, and local levels of government. He worked for the health department of Kansas City, the Missouri Department of Health, and the Centers for Disease Control and Prevention. Malone received his bachelor of arts degree from the University of Illinois at Chicago and his master of public administration degree from the University of Missouri in Columbia.

Deborah Markenson worked for more than 30 years at the Missouri Department of Health and Senior Services in the food, nutrition, and chronic disease control and prevention units. She served at Children's Mercy Hospital as director of collaborative community-based efforts to prevent and treat childhood obesity in the greater Kansas City area. Markenson also formally established a statewide advisory group to provide oversight and to facilitate collaboration between the healthcare, public health, early childhood, school, and academic sectors to prevent and treat childhood obesity.

Allese B. McVay is a program coordinator at the Saint Louis University College for Public Health and Social Justice. She has experience in grant/contract management and public health systems and services research. She has managed multiple National Institutes of Health– and Robert Wood Johnson Foundation–funded grants focusing on dissemination and implementation, neighborhood effects on chronic disease, obesity, and cancer outcomes. McVay holds a master of public health degree from Saint Louis University.

Tapan Mehta, PhD, is an associate professor in the School of Medicine of the University of Alabama at Birmingham (UAB). He is the director of biostatistics and data management core for the UAB/Lakeshore Foundation Research Collaborative.

Kimberly Peeren is director of consulting services at Conduent Healthy Communities Institute, where she manages the development and delivery of services to hospitals, health departments, and collaborative groups in support of their community health improvement efforts. Peeren holds a bachelor's degree in integrative biology and religious studies from the University of California, Berkeley; a master's degree in humanities from San Francisco State University; and a master's degree in public health from the University of California, Los Angeles.

Ciaran Phibbs, PhD, is a health economist at the Department of Veterans Affairs (VA) Palo Alto Health Care System's Health Economics Resource Center. He is also an associate professor of pediatrics (neonatology) at Stanford University and an associate of Stanford's Center for Health Policy and Center for Primary Care and Outcomes Research. At the VA, he is the associate director of the Geriatrics and Extended Care Data and Analysis Center and the Women's Health Evaluation Initiative. Dr. Phibbs's research spans from neonates through older adults and end of life. He holds a PhD in economics from the University of California, San Diego.

James A. Rice, PhD, FACHE, is managing director, governance and leadership, for Gallagher's Human Resources & Compensation Consulting practice. He also serves on the American Hospital Association's Foster McGaw Award Committee to champion community health partnerships. Dr. Rice lectures at the School of Public Health of the University of Minnesota; Strathmore University in Nairobi, Kenya; and Cambridge University in England. As past president of The Governance Institute, he is dedicated to strengthening the performance of health sector boards in North America.

James H. Rimmer, PhD, is a professor in the School of Health Professions at the University of Alabama at Birmingham (UAB), the first Lakeshore Foundation Endowed Chair in Health Promotion and Rehabilitation Sciences at UAB, director of research at the Lakeshore Foundation, and an adjunct professor in the Department of Physical Medicine and Rehabilitation at UAB.

Margaret Rost is a consultant on community health initiatives. Previously, she was the community benefits coordinator at the University of Vermont Medical Center. She provides project management for various community programs, including community benefit and community health needs assessments. She holds a master of public administration degree and is currently pursuing a master of social work degree at Portland State University.

Michael Rozier, PhD, is an assistant professor in the Department of Health Management and Policy at Saint Louis University, with a secondary appointment to the Gnaegi Center for Health Care Ethics. Rozier received a PhD in health services organization and policy from the University of Michigan and an MHS in international health from Johns Hopkins University. He currently serves on the board of directors for SSM Health Corporation. His research focuses on the ethical challenges of population health strategies.

Jim Rudolph, MD, is a professor of medicine and health services, policy, and practice at Brown University. He is an expert on cognitive aging, delirium, the application of evidence-based practices to settings, and long-term care. Dr. Rudolph directs the Providence VA Medical Center's Center of Innovation on Long-Term Services and

Supports. He holds a baccalaureate degree from the University of Illinois, an MD degree from Loyola University, and an MS degree from Harvard University.

Marianne Shaughnessy, PhD, is the director for policy, practice, and population health integration in the Veterans Health Administration (VHA) Office of Geriatrics and Extended Care. She is an adult-gerontological nurse practitioner with more than 30 years of experience in clinical care. Prior to joining VHA, she enjoyed a career in academics, teaching and conducting research with older adults.

Eduardo J. Simoes, MD, is chair of the Department of Health Management and Informatics (HMI) at the University of Missouri School of Medicine. He also holds the title of Dr. Stuart Wesbury and HMI Alumni Distinguished Professor in the department. He received his medical degree from the University of Pernambuco in Brazil, his diploma and master of sciences degree from the University of London School of Hygiene and Tropical Medicine, and his master of public health degree from Emory University. He is a fellow of the American College of Epidemiology.

Katherine A. Stamatakis, PhD, is an associate professor of epidemiology at the Saint Louis University College for Public Health and Social Justice. Her expertise is in chronic disease epidemiology, implementation science, and public health systems research. Her research projects strive to improve understanding of the unequal distribution of health promotion resources and to identify community systems and structures that could be better leveraged to promote health and reduce disparities.

Carleen Stoskopf, ScD, is a professor of health management and policy at San Diego State University (SDSU). She has served as director of the Graduate School of Public Health at SDSU and as chair of the Department of Health Services Policy and Management at the University of South Carolina. Her work has focused on healthcare access, utilization, and outcomes among vulnerable populations. She is also an expert in international health. She received her ScD from Johns Hopkins University.

Kevin Syberg, DrPH, is assistant professor for the Department of Health Management and Policy in the College for Public Health and Social Justice at Saint Louis University.

Ranak Trivedi, PhD, is a clinical and health psychologist and investigator with the US Department of Veterans Affairs Health Services Research and Development Center for Innovation to Implementation in Palo Alto, California, and an assistant professor in the Department of Psychiatry and Behavioral Sciences at Stanford University. Dr. Trivedi focuses on ways in which families and patients can better collaborate to improve health outcomes for both, barriers and facilitators of chronic illness self-management, and assessment and treatment of mental illnesses in primary care settings.

Deryk Van Brunt, DrPH, is CEO of CredibleMind, president of the Healthy Communities Foundation, and associate clinical professor in the School of Public Health at the University of California at Berkeley (UC Berkeley). CredibleMind works to improve the mental health and emotional well-being of communities. The Healthy Communities Foundation has catalyzed web-based technology and services to support hospitals, health systems, local and state health departments, and community collaborations with health improvement strategies. Dr. Van Brunt works with organizations to help them understand the health risks in the communities they serve, meet regulatory requirements, plan best-practice interventions, and build evaluation plans. He received his DrPH in health informatics from UC Berkeley.

Jamie Wade is director of outpatient rehabilitation services and community partnership at UAB Hospital in Birmingham, Alabama. Wade specializes in the treatment of communication issues in the adult population with neurological disorders.

Jillian Warriner is manager for community benefit and health improvement at Sharp HealthCare (Sharp) in San Diego, California. She leads the process of identifying community health needs and developing programs to address those needs for the communities served by Sharp's seven hospitals. She is responsible for community health needs assessment and implementation strategy development for the Sharp system, oversees development of Sharp's annual community benefit report, and plays a key role in partnership development and program management and implementation. She holds a master's degree in public health from San Diego State University, with a focus on health policy and management.

Kristin D. Wilson, PhD, is associate professor in the Department of Health Management and Policy and executive director of the Heartland Center for Population Health and Community Systems Development at Saint Louis University College for Public Health and Social Justice.

Wilma J. Wooten, MD, is the senior public health officer for the County of San Diego. Dr. Wooten is an ardent supporter of public health and has a strong interest in health disparities and health equity. She has exerted a major leadership role in the vision and implementation of Live Well San Diego. Previously, Dr. Wooten practiced medicine as a faculty member in the University of California, San Diego (UCSD), Department of Family and Preventive Medicine. Dr. Wooten received both her master's degree in public health and her medical degree from the University of North Carolina, Chapel Hill, and she completed her residency training at the Georgetown/Providence Hospital Family Practice Residency Program in Washington, DC. She also completed the joint San Diego State University (SDSU) Graduate School of Public Health (GSPH) / UCSD Preventive Medicine Residency, with an emphasis in sports medicine.